Obesity in America,
1850–1939

Obesity in America, 1850–1939

A History of Social Attitudes and Treatment

KERRY SEGRAVE

McFarland & Company, Inc., Publishers
Jefferson, North Carolina, and London

LIBRARY OF CONGRESS CATALOGUING-IN-PUBLICATION DATA

Segrave, Kerry, 1944–
    Obesity in America, 1850–1939 : a history of social attitudes
and treatment / Kerry Segrave.
        p.   cm.
    Includes bibliographical references and index.

    ISBN 978-0-7864-4120-4
    softcover : 50# alkaline paper

    1. Obesity — United States — History —19th century.
2. Obesity — United States — History — 20th century.   I. Title.
[DNLM: 1. Obesity — history — United States.   2. Diet,
Reducing — history — United States.   3. History, 19th Century —
United States.   4. History, 20th Century — United States.
5. Social Perception — United States.   WD   210   S455o   2008]
RC628.S438   2008
362.196'398 — dc22   2008027496

British Library cataloguing data are available

Cover image: ©2008 Shutterstock.

Manufactured in the United States of America

*McFarland & Company, Inc., Publishers
    Box 611, Jefferson, North Carolina 28640
    www.mcfarlandpub.com*

Contents

Preface

This book looks at obesity in America from 1850 to 1939, with particular emphasis on the causes of fatness that were advanced over time, to the stereotypes associated with the condition, to employment issues, and to remedies proposed over time for the condition. The first period, from 1850 to 1879, saw very little attention devoted to obesity, mainly because there was little or no overweight problem at the time. What little there was could be found among the upper class. Even then there was no image of fat as being beautiful; most stereotypes associated with fatness were negative, but not all. As well, there was nothing that could be called a science of obesity then; it was quackery from all quarters, from the quacks to the respectable medical people to the scientific community. Fat men's clubs — little more than an excuse for the overweight to indulge in huge meals — sprang up all over America.

Much more media attention was devoted to obesity in the second period, 1880 to 1919, during which quacks continued to dispense quackery while the respectable medical and scientific communities moved from quackery to a more reasonable and accurate assessment of obesity. For example, that latter group, or at least the majority, declared in the early and middle years of that period that ordinary tap water was fattening. Around the same time the quacks were hyping the somersault cure. However, by the end of this period the idea that obesity was mainly a question of calories in and calories out was starting to take hold, although it was still a minority viewpoint. Evidence of the public interest in obesity could be seen in the well-publicized efforts of U.S. presidents William

Preface

Taft and Grover Cleveland to lose weight, efforts followed closely in the press. It was a period when certain foods were branded as bad, or fattening, with no account taken of caloric value of the items. Most often listed as bad foods were the potato, the banana, and bread. Increasingly the idea was presented during this period that there were many more fat women than there were fat men and articles more and more were written about obesity and women only, in addition to articles on obesity and the general population. Science took over in other ways in this period. Diets and menu plans published in the media began to speak of the caloric value of food items late in the period; height and weight tables and mortality tables were generated from life insurance policyholder data. Obesity was branded as an unhealthful and dangerous state, based for the first time on hard evidence. In the last period covered in this book, 1920 to 1939, the science of obesity came to resemble that which still exists in the 21st century. Strange and bizarre theories were no longer issued by the medical community, almost, with quackery left to the quacks. Calories in and calories out was accepted by this time as the cause of virtually all obesity and that weight loss involved hard work and effort in adjusting that equation through diet and exercise, with diet getting much greater emphasis. Obesity, because of its dangers, was taken up in this period as a public health issue for the first time with various public and private agencies and firms setting up weight reduction programs for their citizens, clients, and employees. Reducing became an even bigger fad among the general population. Based on the amount of media attention devoted to the problem of fat children there were none in America in the period 1850 to 1939. Apparently no media mentions were made prior to 1920 and only about three such items surfaced in the 1920 to 1939 period.

1

Obesity Emerges, Slightly, 1850–1879

There was very little written about obesity in America during the period 1850 to 1879, for several reasons. For one thing, while a national media in the form of newspapers and magazines was in existence it was in a fairly rudimentary form. Along with that the literacy rates were lower than they would be in later decades. An American living in the 1890s was more likely to be literate than his counterpart from the 1860s, and more likely to have a relatively wider access to print media, and to access those publications. Cost of such materials was relatively less in the 1890s, say, than in the 1860s. Another factor was the rise of a wealthy overclass and its increasing spread and influence over time. The capitalist class of the 1860s was only a weak shadow of the robber baron class of the 1890s. That was important because the problems of the ruling class were taken to be the problems of Americans as a whole. And that upper class was more likely to fall victim to fatness than American citizens in general. The wealthy were better able to avoid work and any and all forms of physical exertion that displeased them. Perhaps the most important reason for there being little discussion of obesity in this period, though, was the fact that little of it likely existed. Most Americans lived a life of very hard physical exertion, compared to today, and compared also to the 1920s. It was not easy to become obese. Working against obesity was the food system and food delivery infrastructure of the period. Notably absent were all the packaged and prepared foods that have been such a curse to America, in terms of obesity, especially since the end of World War II. Still, there was some obesity in America during this time, and some mention of ways to achieve weight reduction, and some ideas, mostly bizarre, as to the causes of obesity, albeit that there was no effective science of obesity at the time. Quackery abounded but it was as likely to come from members of the established medical community, as it was to come from quacks. Attitudes toward fat people were mixed but the pairing of obesity with beauty, in a Rubenesque sense, had departed America by 1850, if it had ever arrived.

With 1850 only a few days old the editor of an unnamed western newspaper declared he liked fatness, and indirectly listed many of the stereotypes of the day. "We like fat people — good, jolly, laughing, broad-visaged, honest, fat people.... Fatness is a sign of big health. Fat men are never treacherous — fat women are not sharp tongued — fat boys are not mischievous — fat babies are always good — in fact, fat babies are the kindest, and, therefore the most popular. Commend us to fat people."[1]

Considering fatness as a thoroughly negative condition was the editor of the *Brooklyn Eagle* newspaper in a lengthy article in 1857. He observed, "Plumpness and beauty have often been regarded as inseparable. Siamese twins, from the illustrious regent whose ideal of female loveliness was summed up in 'fat, fair and forty' to the Egyptians who fattened their dames systematically...." After a short preliminary, the editor went on to discuss at length a book written by a Dr. Dancel of Paris in which the idea of whether or not to be fat was treated "as the grand question of human life." Added the editor, "the epitome of welfare is leanness; while the origin of evil, nay, evil itself is fat." He then gave thanks that he was not what could be called stout "For, it appears, it is only a vulgar error to believe that an increase of what is called good plight is any symptom of improving health." And, "the extraordinary development of fat causes first inconvenience, then infirmities, and finally constitutes a malady heretofore considered incurable, and known as obesity."[2]

Next, the editor argued that fatness affected the sexes differently; that for men personal grace was not indispensable to happiness but for women the case was different. Dancel reminded his readers that once women had lost their personal attractions, "their intellectual treasures serve merely to render them just supportable in society. Beware, therefore, ladies, how you grow to fat! And you also, gentlemen for your pockets' sake." In the editor's opinion, fat had ruined the prospects of many a man and many a woman, by rendering it impossible for them to continue in a profession that gave them an honorable livelihood. "The infantry officer, overwhelmed with embonpoint [excessive plumpness or stoutness], cannot follow his regiment; the cavalry officer cannot perform his duty on horseback," explained the editor. "The dramatic artist whose voice or whose personal beauty is as good as a gold mine to the theatre that has engaged him, falls into poverty if an avalanche of tallow clogs the powerful lungs, pads the slender waist, and renders shapeless the graceful arms and legs. Stout rope dancers are soon laid flat on their backs; over-grown game-keepers are only fit for targets to be shot at, as practice by juvenile sportsmen." He argued obesity even affected people who lived by mental labor and who "found their faculties clouded by the increase of the corporeal substance." However, he considered it to be an outrageous idea that a literary man who earned his living by his pen would ever have the time to grow "rotund and ponderous."[3]

The editor of the *Eagle* added that those disadvantages he had already noted were only "slight and few," compared to the health problems generated by embonpoint, which he said was a common cause of sterility in both man and beast. An "excess of fat causes the human epidermis to crack, mottling the skin with white speckles and streaks; it induces hernias of various distressing forms; it is the parent of ulcerated legs; it gives rise to headaches, giddiness, and dimness of sight," he declared. "In short, among the infinity of causes which originate disease, a bloated habit of body takes conspicuous rank, although modern medical works bestow but little notice on this morbid disposition." Noted was that such "evils" were often sought to be remedied by medical personnel by bleeding but he argued, "The palliative bleedings are prodigiously conducive to the development of fat.... The palliative of bleeding, therefore, is only temporary; the more you are bled the sooner you are stricken with apoplectic fat." According to the editor, fat people attacked by apoplexy were almost sure to die, while lean people had a very fair chance of recovery. Among other maladies fat people were prone to were, "Dropsy, swelling of the legs, and incurable sores, are the consequences of fat at the liver. Fat people, too, are liable to skin diseases, and to multitudinous other disfigurements besides."[4]

Six years later in 1863, the *Brooklyn Eagle* returned with another lengthy article on the subject of obesity. Admitting it was difficult to tell how much fat on a body was too much the editor went on to declare, "It is a common prejudice that fat persons are slow of intellect, and the provincial epithet of 'fat head' sufficiently expresses the popular idea of the mental prowess of the corpulent. But there are plenty of instances which conflict with this view; and I need only mention David Hume and Napoleon to convince every one that it is not universally true." After giving a few examples of very fat people who were bright he went on to comment that those examples of muscular and mental activity in very fat people did not prove that fat was no hindrance to body or mind; "on the contrary, I am quite ready to confess that they are exceptions to the general rule. There can be little doubt that, in the majority of instances, the development of a large amount of fat diminishes bodily and mental activity...." The ancient name given to the disease of obesity, he said, was polysarkia (abundance of flesh) and "it is evident that they [medical forefathers] all regarded fatness, in otherwise healthy subjects, as a sign of exuberant life. We can hardly hold such an opinion in these days." In his view there had been a discovery wherein "fatty degeneration," a process by which the more highly organized tissues were degraded to a lower organic type, frequently co-existed with the exuberant formation of adipose tissue. But the more accurate clinical observation, which had taught that fatty subjects as a rule could not well sustain the shock of acute diseases, warned us against that view of the matter, and taught that, other things being equal, we should look with distrust upon the health of an individual who rapidly and without some obvious cause became extremely corpulent. "It is probable that the very fact of a tendency to exuberant fatty formation is itself an indication of a certain constitutional vice by no means on the side of strength."[5]

One positive trait attached to obesity was the idea of a lack of criminality. It was an idea that was expressed from time to time throughout this entire period. A news account from 1865 declared, "It is a notable fact in criminal statistics that no fat man was ever convicted of the crime of murder. Stout persons are not very revengeful, nor, as a general thing, are they agitated by gusts of passions. Few murderers weigh more than ten stones [a stone equals 14 pounds]. There are, however, exceptions which justify us in assuming eleven as the utmost limits of the sliding scale, but beyond that there is no impulse toward homicide." Also, the account stated that seldom had such a phenomenon as a fat housebreaker been paraded at the criminal bar; it was the lean, wiry type that did the housebreaking.

"Corpulence, we maintain, is the outward sign not only of a good constitution, but of inward rectitude and virtue," concluded the report.[6]

A reporter or columnist in 1869 ruminated about a fat conductor on a city tram on the Fulton Avenue line in Brooklyn, who worked his ponderous way through the car. Then the author went on to talk about fat people in general. "I have no prejudice against fat people. On the contrary, I like to see them, they look so jolly and seem to be so happy," explained Corry O'Lanus. "They are so good natured, never get cross or scold the family. Can anything be more comfortable to contemplate than a stout old lady? There is a limit, of course, to size; three hundred and fifty pounds is about heavy enough. There are drawbacks to this enlarged sphere of life in extreme cases." Corry added, "Fat people always seem to do well in the world. You never see a fat man begging. Or grinding a hand organ. Buying up soap fat. Propelling a junk cart. Keeping a sidewalk jewelry store. Or an open air dispensary on the cross walk. No sir, they are always to be found in some respectable business, running a bank, managing a theatre, selling oysters, taking charge of a railroad, keeping a hotel, presiding over all sorts of stock companies and money enterprises." Some of the O'Lanus' article was gently tongue-in-cheek, as when he observed that fat men sometimes went into politics but that he never knew a fat man to run for any office lower than Alderman. Claiming his city's government was run mostly by fat men, he cited the positions of Comptroller, Treasurer, Auditor, and Corporation Counsel, although he did not name those officeholders. "I don't know many fat doctors, but fat lawyers always flourish.... A few very good fat men are admitted to the ministry, and they make very unctuous preachers," he stated. "In domestic life the fat man is generally a success. He never beats his wife — it calls for too much exercise, and people would say he ought to be ashamed of himself on account of his size."[7]

An editorial in the *New York Times* in 1877 began by discussing a proposed new method of propelling ships, from an inventor. Then the editor moved on to satirize fat men as being put to use for that purpose, since they had all that energy. "There is a vast quantity of fat men in the world, and it is painfully evident that they have no clear idea what they are placed here for," he kidded. "The fat man is a mystery to himself, and his vague groping after his correct solution are shown by his practice of associating himself with other fat men in clubs, and performing Herculean feats of public overeating." One trend satirized by the editor was the propensity for fat men to form social clubs for themselves in this period. There were a large number of such organizations. "Professional observers have failed to interpret the true meaning of the fat men's clubs, and have carelessly assumed that they are organized merely to gratify an abnormal desire on the part of fat men to make themselves conspicuously ridiculous," he said. "In reality they are the outward expression of the fat man's vague feeling that he has a mission, and of his noble determination to prove that he was not made without a purpose."[8]

Another aspect of obese people that emerged was the public's fascination with the hugely obese in the form of their display in the "freak" sideshows of the era, usually called dime museums, and occasional stories about such individuals not attached to such public shows. A physician described a case of death from obesity in rural Georgia in 1853. He called the young man, who weighed 565 pounds at the age of 22, "one of the miracles of nature." That young man continued to gain weight until he reached a little over 600 pounds but he was still said to be able to get about with tolerable ease and comfort to himself while he attended to his farm planting chores. Three days prior to his sudden death — at an unstated age but he was probably still in his 20s — he weighed 643 pounds.[9]

According to a very brief news item in 1865 a restaurant had been opened in London, England for fat people where nothing was to be served except food that "checked" obesity. No other details were given.[10]

Dr. Dancel, in his 1850s book, stated there were various causes of obesity. "First, there is the natural disposition and constitutional tendency to fat. Obesity may be hereditary.... Out of every hundred obese persons, ninety have short faces, round eyes, and obtuse or snub noses. It is a fact, therefore, that there are individuals predestined to obesity, whose digestive organs elaborate an extra quantity of fat." According to Dancel, secondary causes of corpulence included "long indulgence in sleep in bed and constant riding in carriages, to the exclusion of walking exercise." Examples he cited to reinforce his theory could be found in "The Bedouin Arab, who is always astir to procure the means of his nomadic existence, is never fat; nor are English husbandmen, who live on a shilling a day, and who earn it.... Oriental ladies who are compelled to stop at home, and also the lady abbesses, of convents, often present extraordinary instance of obesity." Other causes were, a great fondness for farinaceous, starchy and sugary foods; "want of thought, as in manifest in the puffy condition of many idiots; a great absorption of fluids, whether water, beer, tea, or preparations of milk, or by frequent tepid baths, or even by constantly breathing damp air, or such as is slightly surcharged with carbonic acid and deficient in oxygen." Apparently, with every breath of air inhaled and the more oxygen taken in, the more carbon (one of the elements of fat) was thrown off the lungs and consequently from the general system. Thus, "the inhabitant of the clear, pure atmosphere of the mountain, is rarely so fat as the resident in the moister stratum which fills the valley." However, Dancel did state, "But the grand cause of obesity, is our eating and drinking more than enough. It has been said that one of the privileges of the human race is to eat without being hungry and to drink without being dry. This double propensity is found wherever men exist."[11]

Dancel posed the question as to whether it was possible to diminish embonpoint without injuring the health — and replied to his query that it was possible. At that point the *Eagle* editor observed that there existed "professional emaciators" who had attained their result by a surgical operation that consisted in cutting a hole in the patient and taking out his "troublesome lump of fat." There was the story of a rich Pasha who was always accompanied by a traveling surgeon to relieve him of his fat, in that way, as often as it became troublesome. In 1718, a Parisian surgeon named Rhothonet was said to have pioneered such surgery and delivered a noted personage of an enormous paunch; after the operation the patient became slim and active. Rhothonet was reportedly besieged by crowds of people wanting the same relief.[12]

For Dancel, the grand principle to diminish obesity without affecting health was for the patient to live principally on meat, eating only a small quantity of other food and drinking but little (and none of that liquid to be water). The seeker of leanness had to eat very few vegetables, and no rolls, puddings, tarts, potatoes, haricots, pea soup, charlottes, sweet biscuits, apple rolls, or cakes — since all of them had carbon and oxygen for their principle basis. In a hundred parts of human fat there were 79 of carbon, 15 and a fraction of hydrogen, and five and a fraction of oxygen. Water, Dancel explained, was nothing but the protoxide of hydrogen and hydrogen was one of the main elements of fat. If a person persisted in living on "leguminous, farinaceous and liquid diets, he will make fat as certainly as the bee makes honey by sucking flowers." Chemistry explained to Dancel that the principle base of meat was azote, which did not enter into the composition of fat while the principal elements of fruits, sugar, flour, and starch, were carbon and hydrogen, the elements of fat. "Human fat is found ready made in certain aliments which are not flesh, as in olive oil and in all oleaginous seeds. If you live principally on lean meat, you will not fatten so fast as those who follow a regimen composed of carbonic and hydrogenic bases." As evidence he cited carnivorous animals — lions, tigers, and wolves — which were never fat. Louis the 18th was enormously fat, explained the doctor, because of his passion for mealy potatoes.[13]

Means other than diet could be used to take off fat, said Dancel, "overladen sufferers ought to take internally certain substances that aid in the decomposition of fat. The alkalis, for instance, combining with it, form soaps." And, "Soap pills have been prescribed for ages past, to cure obstruction (that is, fat) in the liver. The Vichy waters are recommended for the purpose." It was also the alkali in the Vichy waters that removed the fat. Reportedly a physician named Fleming sometimes succeeded in reducing embonpoint by prescribing soap pills while an English observer spoke highly of alkaline baths as an antidote to obesity. But, warned Dancel, alkalis alone would not deliver a person from their burden of fat if by his diet he took in as many grease-making elements as the alkali drove out. In that case the situation would remain unchanged. "Even when living exclusively on meat you may spoil all by drinking too much," cautioned the French physician. "The absorption of the smallest possible quantity of liquid is an indispensable condition, whether in the form of food, drinks, or baths. A moist atmosphere even encourages the growth of fat; some people become heavier in muggy weather." As a caution he observed that draughts of vinegar and other acids produce leanness (when they did not cause death) only by deranging the general health through the injury they caused the digestive canal. Many young persons were said to have fallen victim to such injury brought on by daily doses of vinegar taken with the object of making themselves thinner. "A persistence in drinking strongly acidulated lemonade as a habitual beverage for the same purpose, has proved scarcely less injurious," Dancel concluded. "As to slight doses of tincture of iodine of potassium, to diminish fat, they may be described in one word — poison."[14]

When the editor of the *Brooklyn Eagle* looked at the question of weight reduction in 1863 he described the truth of the matter as being "tolerably simple. All fatty foods, and, as far as possible, all saccharine and farinaceous matters, should be avoided, including such drinks as contain sugar, dextrin, etc. The total quantity of nourishment taken should be as small as is consistent with health; and its principle items should be lean meat and biscuit. Ordinary bread should be avoided, as also beer and all sweet wine; if any alcoholic drink must be taken, dry sherry, or a little weak spirit and water, would be the most suitable." In this newsman's opinion, obesity could be either the cause of an early death or simply a warning that a tendency to premature decay existed, in which case time was allowed for treatment. He cited Aristotle as having said, "fat persons age early and therefore die early." Things to be most avoided if a tendency to fatness existed, counseled the editor, were "sloth and debilitating influences of all kinds. The former influence is a very serious one. People who tend to be fat are usually not so much inclined to actual sleep as to immobility, retention of one posture for long periods together; and hence they lie in bed, or stand loitering for hours together." Still, he thought that such physical apathy was by no means incompatible with great intellectual activity, but made that outcome more unlikely. "This indolence will hardly fail ultimately to produce a diminution of the respiratory movements and a stagnation of the circulation, and hence, a reduction of the activity of the brain, by reason of the blood which supplies that organ being imperfectly oxygenated." Another complicated relationship, in his view, existed between the amount of fat in the body and the state of the person's nervous system. "On the one hand, it seems certain that indulgence in grief, anxiety, overweening passions of any kind, is almost incompatible with any considerable degree of corpulence," he explained. Partly that was due to the effect of those emotional states in depressing the appetite. "On the other hand, pure intellectual activity has often been seen in corpulent persons; according to my experience, such persons are large eaters.... My own opinion certainly inclines to the belief that hard brain workers require rather more than less of easily assimible fat if they have an irresistible tendency to corpulence than if they are lean, supposing that there is no serious defect in the digestion in either case," the editor concluded.[15]

An 1871 article from *Hall's Journal of Health*, excerpted in a newspaper, told the story of a 70-year-old who thought he was too fleshy "and began to Bantingize." He lost 10 pounds in 10 weeks but then developed a medical problem; its exact nature was unstated but the implication was that it came about as a direct result of following Banting's weight reduction plan. William Banting, 1797–1878, was an English undertaker and dietician whose diet plan became so popular that his name came to be used as a verb, as the question, for example, "are you banting?" came to refer to his method and to dieting in general. He was one of the first people to go on what we today call a low-carbohydrate diet plan. Banting was 64 years old in 1861, and 5'5" in height and weighed 202 pounds when he began his diet, after trying almost everything then being touted to produce a weight loss. Several months later he was down to 156 pounds. Later in that decade he declared his diet plan a success and published a booklet on the method that sold very well. Under his system he gave up items such as bread, butter, milk, sugar, beer, and potatoes, while being allowed meat of any kind (except pork, which was then thought to contain starch). Banting ate a high-protein diet with both carbohydrates and fats restricted, and with no limitations of the quantity of food consumed. For decades his name and diet plan were cited, both for condemnation and commendation, as he remained the figure most closely identified with diet plans in the American mind. According to the medical journal, "If a man can sleep soundly, has a good appetite, with no unpleasant reminders after meals, the bodily habits being regular every day, he had better let himself alone, whether he be as big as a hogshead or as thin and dry as a fence rail." Several cases of Bright's disease were said to be "a direct result of practicing Banting's plan for getting lean. The very best and safest way to get rid of fat is to work it off. This may be aided by eating food which contains a large amount of nitrogen and a small amount of carbon." Nitrogen foods — such as lean meats — were said to give strength and power to work while "carboniferous" foods such as cheese, potatoes, rice, corn, peas, beans, tapioca, arrowroot, cornstarch, milk, sugar, syrup, and all oily and fat foods, were those that made fat. The writer of this article commended the eating of large amounts of raw fruits and berries as great aids to reducing weight and concluded, "But, after all, the great reliance should be on exercise and work in the open air." Especially mentioned was walking.[16]

An 1866 article from the same medical journal proclaimed, "Great eaters never live long" and that a voracious appetite, far from being a sign of health, was a certain indication of disease. "Multitudes measure their health by the amount they eat; and out of ten persons, nine are gratified at an increase of weight; when in reality an excess of fat is, in proportion, decisive proof of disease, showing that the absorbents of the system are too weak to discharge their duty; and the tendency to fatness, to obesity, increases until existence is a burden, and sudden death closes the history," declared the piece. Particular inquiry, it continued, would almost always elicit the fact that fat persons, "however rubicund and jolly, are never well, and yet they are envied ... small eaters — those who eat regularly of plain food — usually have no spare flesh, are wiry and enduring and live to an active old age."[17]

A news account in 1870 observed, "It has been said all the flesh and all the fat we ever gain is accomplished during sleep. There is, no doubt, some truth in this remark. The infant is usually fat, and he sleeps the greater part of the time. The fat person, also, sleeps very much. Old persons sleep but little, and when this season comes, as it does with by far the larger part, they begin to lose the rotundity of body, which characterized them at middle life, and, as the common expression is, 'dry up.'" It caused the reporter to conclude that if a person desired to lose fat and become thin, he should sleep but little as "This will reduce obesity faster than any other means can." More generally, he concluded, "The best remedy for obesity is, keep cool by day and night, sleep little, moderate indulgence in eating and drinking, and plenty of exercise. Whoever will observe these rules will not likely become too fat. Some kinds of food produce more fat than others; nothing is more fattening than Indian meal."[18]

An anecdotal account of the prevalence of fat women — and likely exaggerated — came in a dispatch from Saratoga, New York, in 1875, when the place enjoyed the status of being a very fashionable summer resort for the wealthy class. "And so many fat women! We begin to think there is an exhibition of them on hand — something after the fashion of a baby show. There are fat women to the left of us, fat women to the right of us, fat women to the front of us, and fat women to the back of us, until they must reach the 'six hundred' of Tennyson's Light Brigade at Balaklava," went the account. It continued, "the more flesh they carry about the more they adorn it; and the fat women bear off the palm in conspicuous dressing. Great diamonds nestle in folds of fat, and rest on bunches of flesh like the velvety cushions that jewelers display in their showcases...."[19]

For other observers, though, the obese people were elsewhere. When a Dr. Giles of Manhattan was touting an anti-fat remedy he declared, "the most marked peculiarity that will impress the American traveler when he walks the streets of London [England] for the first time is the great number of excessively fat people whom he everywhere meets." As he continued he brought up the issue of class, "He at first supposes these persons to belong to the nobility, on the same principle that he would pronounce them aldermen or bankers if seen in Boston or New York. In brief, he labors under the popular though mistaken impression, that obesity is invariably the combined result of laziness and high living; while in reality it is a constitutional disease."[20]

An 1879 news report discussed the idea that there was a "popular though erroneous notion that health is synonymous with fat." In the opinion of this account, obesity was "an abnormal condition of the system, in which the saccharine and oleaginous elements of the food are assimilated to the partial exclusion of the muscle-forming and brain-producing elements. In proof of this it is only necessary to assert the well-known fact that excessively fat people are never strong, and seldom distinguished for mental powers or activity. Besides, they are the easy prey of acute and epidemic disease, and they are the frequent victims of gout, heart disease and apoplexy."[21]

Clubs for fat men abounded in this period. They were social in nature and concerned themselves mostly with annual balls, annual summer picnics, and so forth. Membership was generally open only to men who weighed 200 pounds or more, which was about as close as one got to a working definition of "fat" in this period. On the evening of November 24, 1869, 3,098 pounds "of well-dressed flesh, or thirteen members [average weight of 238 pounds]" of the Fat Men's Association of New York City met at the Revere house hotel to arrange matters for a ball to be given by them at Irving Hall in the following month. That organization had only recently formed and was one of the first, or perhaps the first, such club in America.[22]

One month later, on December 20, the first annual ball of the organization was held. By then it had a reported 150 to 200 members, with members being required to weigh no less than 200 pounds. According to a news report, at the ball "The fair partners of the fat terpsichoreans were, as a general thing, slim waisted and slender, which shows that the Association pays due regard to the law of compensation. There were enough heavyweights, however, among the sex to vindicate the theory of women's rights and prove that women can compete with men, even in fatness, if they choose." The fattest man present was J. A. Fiske, president of the group, who weighed 358 pounds. A further description from an attending reporter said, "The dancing, or rather the ponderous movement of the Titans, commenced at 9:30 o'clock in the evening and was kept up until 2 or 3 in the morning [and was] performed with as much regularity and conscientious zeal, as if dancing were the natural avocation of fat men instead of a grotesque attempt to defy nature." And, when supper was served at 11:30 P.M., "the fat men found themselves at home, and joined heartily in their devotions to the voracious deity from whom they derived their inspirations and their fat.... Altogether it was an elegant affair."[23]

At that time the city of Brooklyn had among its residents, some members of the Fat Men's Association of New York and, according to a reporter, many others of note who were understood to be candidates. Existing members were, Frank Swift (contractor, 251 pounds), John S. Bogart (Superintendent of the Brooklyn Water Works, 255), Henry Palmer (Superintendent of the Brooklyn City Railroad, 266), Alderman Moses H. Richards (11th Ward, 236), and Mark Phraner (Inspector of Sewers, 219). Some of those mentioned as candidates were; Francis McNeeley (Keeper of the Kings County Penitentiary, 260), Sam Bedell (Inspector of Water Pipes, 280), former alderman Louis Newman (225), and four others, each above 211 pounds. Additionally, the reporter named a few others that he called notable Brooklyn heavies, Grenville T. Jenks (lawyer, 312), Louis Van Pelt Post (private watchman, 400), John Beatty (sergeant in the NYPD, 41st Precinct, 240, known sarcastically to felons as "Slim Jim"), Dr. George Cochran (police surgeon, 230), Albert Weeks (offered a new suit of clothes if he would go to New York and be initiated into the club, estimated at 500 pounds), Captain Smith (NYPD, 42nd Precinct, 231), Captain Brown (NYPD, 48th Precinct, 237).[24]

A year later, in June 1870, it was reported that the German Fat Men's Association of New York went on an excursion and picnic. Many of the members were listed by name and by weight with the two biggest being Adam Brandt (286 pounds) and Max Spraul (258). Among the guests was J. A. Fiske, still 358 pounds, who invited the German fat men to a clambake arranged by his own group for later in that year. Said a reporter, "The dancing of the fat men was of course very graceful, although, especially when they danced with fat ladies, of whom several were present, they circumscribed pretty large circles."[25]

The United Association of the Heavy Men of New York State held its first annual clambake on August 19, 1870. It was an offshoot, said a journalist, "of the famous Fat Men's Association [of New York] whose existence and general hospitality are well known to all." Organized in January 1870 it then had some 125 members. Although members would not give their individual weights to a reporter, he declared, "Collectively, however, they were very desirous of being considered as heavy in every way."[26]

During the summer of 1872 invitations went out for the "Annual Convention of Fat Men" to be held at Put-in-Bay Island, Ohio, on September 10, 1872. The circular for the event stated, "The hotels on the island have agreed that special efforts shall be made to make the visit a pleasant one, and no pains will be opened by the committee in charge of this event of the season. All parties weighing 200 pounds and over will be permitted to deliberate with the convention." Speeches, lectures, readings, recitations, whistling, wrestling, jumping, racing, rowing, fishing, swimming, singing, dancing, eating, drinking, and so on, constituted the amusement for the event. The heaviest man present at the convention was to be named president of the group for the coming year. At that convention addresses on obesity, its causes and cures, were given by "celebrated" physicians. But the real highlight of the affair, and at most such gatherings of fat men's groups was the clambake — that is, the portion of the program that featured much eating.[27]

The sixth annual clambake of the Fat Men's Association of New York was held on August 27, 1874. Prior to the dinner an official weighing of the members took place — and was a common feature at many such gatherings of fat men's societies. Forty-eight names and weights of individuals were listed in a newspaper account, with the total weight of that group being 11,844 pounds, an average of 246.7 pounds. The three largest members were, W. A Lewis (532 pounds), Willard Perkins (369), and W. J. Jacoy (351). Altogether 96 people over 200 pounds were weighed; a total of 21,527 pounds, or an average of 224.5 pounds.[28]

When the Fat Men's Association held its annual clambake in 1877 it reportedly had 300 members. The names and weighs of 15 men weighing over 250 pounds were given (four of them weighed over 300 pounds each). Leading the way was Willard Perkins who was then up to 399 pounds.[29]

Yet another such group was the Heavy Weights, a society organized for the express purpose of eating clams and chickens, and a group said to have had its 13th annual clambake at Taylor's Hotel in Pleasant Valley, New Jersey, on September 4, 1879. No other details of the group were given except, noted a reporter, "They have reached the proportions of members of the Fat Men's Assoc."[30]

2

Psychology and Effects, 1880–1919

The period 1880 to 1919 saw a huge increase in interest in the topic of obesity with a great many more articles in the media devoted to it. Columnists, both medical and lay, offered advice to the general public on being overweight and what could be done about it. There were just as many fat men's clubs as before and fat men's races at various field days and large, organized picnics became common. For the first time attention was paid to obesity in the workplace where it was not always seen as harmless or viewed with bemusement. Especially mentioned in job-related discussion was one of the more enduring stereotypes that sprang mostly from this time — that of the fat cop. Ideas and advice on causes and cures of obesity, diets, and how to reduce abounded with a transition taking place. At the beginning of the period quackery continued to dominate with science a distant second. However, by the end of World War I the scientific arguments on obesity began to hold sway. Quackery, of course, did not disappear, but more and more it came only from the quacks, not the medical establishment.

There was even an article in defense, to some extent, of obesity. According to an 1880 piece in the London, England, medical journal *The Lancet,* "it is unpleasant to be excessively obese; but the morbid dread of fat which has in recent years become fashionable, has no foundation in physiological fact." Fat was said to serve two purposes: it acted as an envelope for the body and protected it from a too rapid loss of heat; and it served as a store of fuel. Also noted was that in the course of exhausting diseases it not infrequently happened that the life of a patient was prolonged while the reserve of fat was exhausted. Fats supplied the material of the heating process on which vitality mainly depended. "In great excess it is inconvenient, but the external layings-on-of-fat is no certain measure of the internal development of adipose tissue; much less does a tendency to grow fat imply or even suggest a tendency to what is known as 'fatty degeneration,'" added *The Lancet*. And, "It is time to speak out on this point, as the most absurd notions seem to prevail. Again, it is not true that special forms of food determine fat. This is an old and exploded notion."[1]

In 1883 a reporter observed that an examination of police records for almost any city in America would show that where "one fat person falls into the hands of the police upward of one dozen lean persons share the same fate." He went on to add that American girls of the time "not withstanding the fact that they are very much addicted to a too liberal use of the corset, and in fact, in many cases to a superlative degree, deem it necessary to make use of acids (foods such as vinegar and lemons) in order to prevent obesity. If they would forego the use of acetic matter and indulge in rational amounts of exercise they would find it far more beneficial to the development of their forms and conducive to health." In his opinion it was a general error to suppose that men or women of genius did not become fat and that all poets had to become lean and melancholy. Examples of fat, bright men he cited were Balzac ("exceedingly stout"), the composer Rossini ("another of the Jumbo race of celebrities"), the elder Dumas, and Lord Byron and Eugene Sue, "both dreaded their tendency to fatness and were known to indulge frequently in vinegar and lemons and other acids." Even then, he pointed out, stage actors both male and female always feared their careers would come to a sudden end if they became obese. Reportedly, the then late Mrs. John Brougham was compelled to quit the stage "on account of the extra rotundity of her form, although in her young days she was always selected to represent the sylph-like characters." His conclusion was, "There is no doubt that fatness can be cured by a strict adherence to a system of moderation in gastronomic matters...and by indulging in a good five mile walk upon each pleasant day of the year."[2]

That same year one of the stereotypes of fat men was presented in a humorous, satirical article about obese men sleeping in Pullman railroad cars. On the trains the lower berths were more popular with all travelers than were the upper berths and, as a result, were always booked up first. Stories circulated widely about fat men in upper berths crashing through their accommodation and injuring people asleep in lower berths. Although such an incident had never occurred, that fact did not prevent the stories making the rounds. According to one journalist, a well-known (but unnamed) New York reporter who weighed 300 pounds was the originator of the story. If that man reached a train late and all the lower berths were taken he then worked a joke with a porter who was in on the deception. Standing near the lower berth the fat man wanted he would ask the porter how Mr. Smith was and the porter would say oh, you mean the guy who suffered a broken rib and arm when you crashed through from your upper berth onto him, and so on.[3]

If Rubenesque stature was once revered such was not always the case in the ancient past. As long ago as the days of the Greeks and Romans, a slight figure was admired and stoutness was looked upon as a deformity, according to an 1884 account. Martial was said to have ridiculed fat women and Ovid put large waists in the first rank of his remedies against love.[4]

An 1885 report remarked that the time was when Sophie Croizette (a famed actor of the period) "then lithe and supple as a panther, was Sarah Bernhardt's most powerful rival, and the adored of all Paris." She was born in St. Petersburg, the daughter of a ballet dancer mother; her grandfather was an actor and a playwright. Despite her theatrical background Sophie was educated to be a governess. Then she met an old actress who turned her toward the stage. Two years later she made her debut on the stage in Paris; it was a debut that made her a sensation. "Croizette's fame was established, and she would have been still on the boards had she not suddenly began to grow stout. It was a terrible mishap," said a journalist. "She practiced banting; it was of no avail. She compressed herself into all kinds of fearful and wonderful corsets: they made no difference. She tried quack medicines; they were useless. Not all the patent syrups of the world could ever medicine her to that slim waist which she owned yesterday. Fatal disaster! Catastrophe irreparable! As an actress she was ruined." One of the original fat person gibes went back to the time of Croizette because "It was originally of Croizette that a disappointed admirer said it tired him to make love to her, it took so long to walk round her." As compared to, "Paris screamed over the story that Sarah [Bernhardt] had nearly lost her life by pulling out the stopper in her bath and going down the waste pipe with the water." In the recent years before 1885 it was said "Croizette has acted but little. Her increased fat has rendered her unwieldy, and now her marriage with a wealthy banker is the signal of her withdrawal from the Francais [theater]."[5]

A story in American newspapers in 1886, reprinted from the United Kingdom's *Pall Mall Gazette*, argued the Eastern and Western worlds held different views on the subject of corpulence. In China, it was said, corpulence was considered to be one of the most important qualifications for the holding of any public office. It was regarded as a physical virtue that lent dignity to the appearance, weight to the judgment, and solidity to the mind. Also, in China, "the thin man is always moody and disappointed...Banting, except as a punishment for great criminals is unknown in China. The most popular gods in the Chinese Pantheon are those remarkable for their obesity." Comparing that to Europe the writer of the piece exclaimed how different it was. Cited as a defining difference was the situation of Daniel Lambert (a famous fat man in the West who weighed, reportedly, over 700 pounds, and was prominently on public display in the dime museums — in the parlance of the day a "freak" in a "freak show"). The Chinese, thought the reporter, would have sent the likes of Lambert to a province as a mandarin, while in the West he was sent to a museum as a monstrosity. Also cited was Byron's tendency to grow fat being one of the causes of his melancholy, "and the declining years of the first gentleman in Europe were rendered miserable by that stoutness which even stays could not conceal." Shakespeare intended Hamlet to be fat, said the account, "feeling probably that it would be characteristic of such a lethargic nature, but modern audiences are not ready to accept fat Hamlets: they prefer thin Hamlets, and even lean Hamlets, and seem to be of the opinion that there is an artistic discord between romance and rotundity. And, indeed, it cannot be doubted that this opinion is very widespread..." [6]

One example of the stereotypes and images connected to fat people could be found in a brief editorial in the *Dallas News* in 1891, and reprinted in other papers. "The fat shoat, the fat dog, the fat tom cat, the fat billy goat, are wholly without self-reliance, have no object in life, keep no move on them, can't sing, can't fight — have in them nothing on earth except food which their masters have put there. Let us be lean and independent."[7]

For one journalist in 1893 there were two kinds of women in the world who were morbidly unhappy from what they chose to regard as nature's injustices to them. Those two types were those who were either excessively thin or who were "burdened with an excess of flesh. The former, however, though it may be treason to expose their little frauds, may help nature out by sundry pads and fluffy style of dressing, but the stout woman, despite all her efforts to hide her undue corpulence, is conscious always that her flesh is unwieldy."[8]

From a 1905 article in the *Los Angeles Times* it was learned that two fat holdup men stopped a youth after he left a streetcar, followed him, and then fired shots at the youth after he got wise to the situation and tried to run away. Those shots fired caused him to stop with the holdup men getting small change. In keeping with the idea that obese men were not felons the surprised journalist remarked, "Fat holdup men are something of a novelty, and the police felt inclined at first to doubt the boy's story, but investigation leads to the belief that his assertions are true."[9]

Going against the grain a year later was an unnamed Parisian writer who insisted it was the fat people who should be regarded with the most suspicion. He had just written a book to prove that an abundance of adipose tissue, in male or female, "far from indicating a frank, honest, generous disposition, often serves as a mask for rascality and cunning." Cited as evidence were various examples from contemporary French criminal files. Not only were fat folks more likely to be dishonest than thin ones, but also their obesity made it easier for them to perpetuate frauds, according to the French author. That, he continued, was because of the mistaken notion that rotundity of figure was an indication that its possessor had a clear conscience, it was the result of dealing dishonestly with one's stomach. On the other hand the lean person was "naturally" less disposed to be dishonest and because of the suspicion that his slim figure aroused, found it harder to carry out financial swindles on a large scale.[10]

In 1909 a New York newspaper declared that "Happy is the nation whose magistrate is weighty," going on to imply that stout men were usually both active and good-natured, and then observed that when one looked at contemporary rulers and those who had ruled in the past they were mostly all fat. It was a sentiment seconded by an editor of the *Washington Post*. One example cited was Armand Fallieres, chief magistrate of the French Republic, "a man of voluminous girth and of unalterable good nature."

The late Queen Victoria was described as "extremely stout" as was King Edward. Also, it was reported the only two rulers of Russia whose deaths were known to have been attributable to natural causes, without any positive knowledge or strong suspicion of violence, namely Alexander III and Catherine the Great, "were both persons of extremely heavy build." To the writer of the piece, the fact that in each case their end was peaceful showed that whatever Western nations may have thought about their rule and character, they had the affection and goodwill of their countrymen. Still, he went on to admit there were exceptions to the rule, cases where "the excellence of the character of the sovereign has not been in keeping with their ponderosity." Thus, neither Isabella II of Spain nor her mother the late Queen Christina "can be said to have been good queens, or even reputable sovereigns. Yet they were enormously fat women" and the most obese "monster" within the last hundred years was Louis XVIII of France who, toward the end of his reign, became so heavy that his legs could no longer support his body and he had to be wheeled about in a chair."[11]

Another satirical column about fat men came from the pen of Alma Whitaker in 1913; she was a columnist of long-standing with the *Los Angeles Times*. "The clerical gentleman who recently assured the world that fat men were nearly always virtuous and that tall, thin men were mostly sinful was simply toadying to the bishops, who are mostly plumpish." Then she kidded by saying the question of the relative harmlessness of avoirdupois in the male of the species was a most important issue to poor defenseless women, "and I beg to state calmly and in my right mind that fat men are dangerous." One could tell that from the fact that the fat men secured the handsomest wives. And that despite the fact that virtually all women started out by picturing Prince Charming as slim. "Yet these seductive, devilishly attractive, short, fat men wheedle their way with diabolical cleverness into their sentimental young hearts and before she realizes where she is Imogene, tall, stately and angelic, is wedded to Edward, five-foot-four and turning the scale at 200 pounds." One of the reasons for that outcome was, "it is a sad fact that fat men are the lightest and springiest on their feet as well as in their conversation."[12]

Blanche Beacon argued in a 1914 article that it was a strange thing but she had noticed that thin women were much more aware of their "painful" thinness than were fat women of their "beauty-effacing" fat. She thought, "It may be because the fat woman is the comfortable one of tradition and her lack of worry helps her flesh to accumulate."[13]

The idea that fat people were unpopular was expressed forcefully in 1914 by a reporter who declared, "The slim figure is in the ascendancy. Even the great of the earth cannot afford altogether to disregard the dictates of the fashion which decrees that all men and all women shall present to the world the outlines of spare severity," in a piece reprinted in American papers after appearing originally in the London *Saturday Review*. So powerful was the sway of that sentiment, said the article, that the German kaiser Wilhelm II and former U.S. president William Taft "have both found it necessary to go in for a process of weight reduction." And, "Fat is now regarded as an indiscretion, and almost as a crime. Only the very strong-minded dare to be fat at all, and there are few indeed who glory in corpulence." However, he argued it had not always been so with the 18th century, especially, seeming "to run to over-nourishment. Ruminative repletion in the prevailing expression in the portraits of the period; and the majestic swagger of corpulence is visible in the rolling periods of Gibbons, Burke, Johnson and the rest..." It was a tradition he believed that lasted well into the 19th century with Charles Dickens nearly always treating the fat man — at least the benevolent fat man — with an affectionate respect. "His Pickwick and Cheerybles seem to reflect the conviction that stoutness is not only a natural but a rather laudable condition for the elderly. And when [Dickens' character] Tony Weller declared that 'vidth and visdom go together' he was merely condensing into an epigram the very common English idea that native sagacity was to be found in alliance with a profile of pronounced convexity." But all that was in the past, he concluded; "now the fat man has no defenders. The medical man denounces him. The tailor only makes him a suit under protest. The novelist gives him no question. The dramatist will allow him no more benevolent parts; he is only introduced to look foolish. The labor cartoonist adopts him as a type of the capitalist."[14]

Don P. Smith, a marketing man with the firm of Earl V. Armstrong Inc., studied, in 1916, why certain people bought certain kinds of automobiles and determined it came down to the physical characteristics either of the person or the car. For example, a long-legged person chose a car with plenty of room to stretch out his long legs while "The man with a tendency toward obesity prefers a car with a high steering wheel and deeply upholstered cushions. Adjustable pedals he demands, for comfort with him is the prime requisite."[15]

And then there were the traits and characteristics associated with obesity in this period. "It is generally supposed that fat people have much more blood than others. On the contrary, they have less," explained one writer in 1887. Not only that, but the blood they had was "really poor, while the fat fills the space which is required even for the circulation of that. Fat people have, then, less vital energy than the thin, not possessing sufficient blood to bring every organ up to its full working power, and the fat hindering what blood there is from flowing freely enough to the organs, especially at the moment of action requiring it." In addition, it was explained, that obstructed the working of the lungs so that sufficient air could not be inhaled to purify the blood with the result the natural and necessary combustion was so interfered with that the functions of the body were hindered. "It follows that too much exertion should always be guarded against in people of large and fatty development, and too much should never be expected of them," the article concluded.[16]

A year later an article dealt with the topic of fat men's traits in a tongue-in-cheek manner, but also displayed some of the prevalent images. With respect to obese men in politics, said the piece, "In office fat men serve as ballast to the ship of state. They are always conservative. They believe in old ways. They are cautious and averse to trying dangerous experiments. They will not adopt anything that has not been tested." And, in a more general sense, "They are not likely to overdo anything, except eating and sleeping. They believe in going to bed early and in making up for it by getting up late. They are regular in their habits, one of which is being ready when there is a call for dinner. They are never in a hurry." A man weighing 117 pounds would make more of a disturbance at any sort of meeting, he argued, than would ten men, each of whom weighed 356 pounds.[17]

A journalist asserted in 1890, "It is rather hard for the majority of people to associate intellect with fat, yet some of the greatest men the world has ever known were plump even to obesity." His examples cited were Napoleon, Doctor Johnson and his biographical shadow Boswell, and Balzac who was "so large that it was a pretty bit of exercise to walk around him." Rossini, the composer, who "for six years never saw his knees"; Jules Janin, "the prince of critics, broke every sofa he ever sat upon;

his cheeks and chin protruded beyond his beard and whiskers." And, there was the Italian singer, Lablanche, who "was charged three fares when he traveled," the elder Dumas, Sainte Beuve, and Eugene Sue, who had such an aversion to his growing corpulence that he drank vinegar in an attempt to keep it down.[18]

Writing in the *Hartford Courant* in 1891, a reporter declared, "It is a wide-spread popular error which teaches that fatness is a blessing...But personal superabundance of flesh is to be lamented. History and science alike testify to this." Scholars told us, he continued, that Shakespeare's Hamlet was fat and scant of breath, leading to his "strange indecision in the righteous act of letting the life out of his uncle the dastard king." It meant to the article writer that a man handicapped by fatness was robbed of the energy and quickness necessary to prompt, vigorous action. Science, he argued, said that fatness was a disease and in thinness there is strength. And, one of the more exasperating features of the situation was that all through his life the fat person lost the most precious of human comforts — sympathy. When an obese friend waddled downtown some morning suffering "a hundred present twinges and prospectively suffering neuralgia, fatty degeneration of the heart, gout, apoplexy and a lot more of the ills peculiar to his condition...Why everybody who meets him congratulates him on his splendid appearance, he was never looking so well in his born days; it is invigorating just to see him from across the street [which is easy because of his size]; he will outlast all his relatives." Such talk continued on and if the fat person interrupted to say he wasn't feeling that well, that he slept poorly, and so on, his remarks were received with "amiable skepticism. He might just as well lie about it, for all the pity he gets." With regard to the fat lover, the journalist observed, he "is a monstrosity in literature and hardly to be tolerated in actual life. He of big girth and short wind, when he is in violent motion, provokes the laughter of both gods and men." Not to mention that the obese were shut out of sports and exercise without number. When it came to obese women, "needless to say that the misfortune of obesity spoils their figures, makes dancing an impossible delight and drives them to the banting process to recall their sometimes grace and agility, which blows are harder to bear than the accompanying aches and pains."[19]

Satire and "sport" directed at U.S. President Grover Cleveland's obesity was declared by an 1893 newspaper account to be in "exceedingly bad taste. He may be a gold bug and a Mugwump, but he is not to blame for the huge mountains of fat which sizzle within and around his person. Such a man is to be pitied."[20]

It was reported two years later that President Cleveland received from 10 to 20 letters in the mail each day from the public containing remedies and tips for reducing obesity.[21]

According to an unnamed physician in 1893, fat people endured most kinds of illness much better than did thin people, because they had an extra amount of nutriment stored away in their tissues to support them during the ordeal. Moreover, there were said to be many other consolations for persons of "abundant girth. They are generally optimists by nature, genial and jolly companions, whose society is universally preferred to that of people with angular frames and dispositions."[22]

According to one 1896 journalist there had been a number of notable women of the world, famous not only for their beauty but also for their intellect and "subtle fascination." Women who had helped make history and been a power in their day and "were of distinctly generous proportions." Named were Cleopatra "small and stout" and Marie Antoinette "of the plump order." In the current time were Queen Victoria of England, Queen Margherita of Italy, and Queen Isabella of Spain. "It is worthy of note that most of the great interpreters of song are stout, or bordering on that condition, and there have been lights in the literary world decidedly fat." Cited were Mme. De Steel and George Sand, "fat and small." Despite that, the reporter agreed, "fashion's votaries will doubtless continue to strive after the slenderness which seems so desirable."[23]

Articles declaring that corpulent geniuses were not rare turned up off and on over time for decades. A 1904 piece that appeared originally in a London, England publication mentioned the usual suspects. One problem with those pieces was that almost every one of them mentioned the same small number of people and when looked at as a group tended to reinforce the conclusion that each article denied — that fat geniuses were indeed rare. This piece cited Rossini, and used the same joke that he had not seen his feet (instead of knees) in years, Jules Gabriel Janin, Balzac, and Victor Hugo. The same joke was used about Janin — that he broke all the sofas. Of Balzac it was said three ordinary persons, stretching their hands, could hardly reach around his waist. Politicians mentioned were Germany's Prince Bismarck and the United Kingdom's Lord Salisbury and

Lord Rosebery with those three said to lend support to the idea that "fat men are, as a rule, clever." Judges, he added, almost without exception, were overweight.[24]

Another article from a UK publication, in 1906, spoke about fat as applied to the treatment of mental disease. It appeared that the more the men defined as mentally afflicted were fattened up the saner they became. But the difficulty was said to lie in providing the lunatic with adipose tissue as there was "nothing like brain disease to cause too solid flesh to melt." Reflecting on the attempts people made to reduce, "We bathe, we massage, we diet, we fly to these and those waters, we try all manner of cures and put ourselves into various kinds of straps and pastes and take violent exercise with the aim of slimming ourselves down and keeping stoutness at bay," the writer of the article wondered what it meant with respect to his sanity finding. "Does this decided disposition on the part of men and women to avoid corpulence and the successful thinning down that we notice on all sides portend an increase of lunacy," he wondered?[25]

According to a Mrs. Scanlon, in 1907, it was a "universal rule" that wives of successful men were fat. If they were not, it was proof that they did not love their husbands. A fat girl, added Scanlon, "has all the best of the thin, willowy creature in showiness, in disposition and in temperament." Criticizing obesity remedies, she argued that to be happy women had to be fat. Scanlon explained, "The reason is plain. The wives of the successful men are fat because they are not worried about the next month's rent and the children's clothes. People who pity fat women simply show their ignorance; women who complain because they are stout make themselves unhappy when they should be the happiest women on earth."[26]

Arguing that fat men were not really jolly was a 1908 article in which the reporter declared we had learned the adage, "Laugh and grow fat" was not true. And that we had come instead to a slow realization that fat was a very dangerous disease and not a state of giggling happiness. Many fat people, he said, laughed in public "just as a safety valve to their misery and to make us believe that their smiles are genuine. Some are really jolly, but not because they are fat. To most of the jolly ones as well as to the others, every coming and going of their breath is a puff of misery and their smiles are sadder than the tears of childhood."[27]

An unnamed "fat gentleman" spoke up in a 1908 *Washington Post* article and defended his brethren. In particular he spoke in praise of some fat politicians, namely Daniel Webster, "broad in body as well as in mind," Judah P. Benjamin, formerly a Senator from Louisiana and later the Attorney General of the Southern Confederacy. Additionally, he cited Stephen A. Douglas as having corpulence and brains, the late Speaker Reed, ex-president Grover Cleveland, and Secretary William Taft. The author of the piece admitted there were some fat men who wanted to be thin but "They are in a majority of cases, however, candidates for museum honors, and they are few and far between." After asserting that great personal bulk and chivalry were almost always found together, he concluded, "It may afford you some solace also to know that there are more female specimens of remarkable obesity than in the opposite sex. The ordinary fat man who mingles daily with the world is a comfort to himself and a pride to his friends."[28]

The supposed connection between weight and literary genius was commented on by Robert Sherard in his *Modern Paris* in 1914. Among the usual suspects he named were Balzac, "always fat and jolly," Alexandre Dumas, Rossini, Victor Hugo and Sainte Beuve. As well he cited Theopile Gautier, an "enormous" man who maintained that a man of genius should be fat, and Emile Zola, said to have written best when he was very stout and that when his bulk dwindled, so did his talent. Byron was mentioned and some detail given of the freak diets he tried in an effort to control his increasing bulk that he found so disagreeable. In 1813 Byron lived on six biscuits a day and tea; "Don Juan" was written almost entirely on gin and water, and while at Athens he tried a diet of rice in small quantities washed down by vinegar and water.[29]

The *Washington Post* published a 1916 article, from a UK publication, listing fat men of genius noting that "It is frequently averred that fat is deadening to the brain, and consequently a foe to intellectual activity," before mentioning Napoleon, Dr. Johnson, Boswell, Balzac, Janin, Rossini, and Victor Hugo.[30]

"Laugh and grow fat" had been a proverb for hundreds of years, according to a reporter in 1916, adding, "Jolliness and stoutness are generally found together; not that all stout people are jolly but that nearly all jolly people are stout." The reason for that, he argued, was physiological, with fat being the result of good digestion. "It shows that the food eaten is readily changed by the processes of the body into living tissue," he explained. "Of course, extreme stoutness or obesity may become so inconvenient as almost to be a disease, but, even so, this is still due to the ability of the body to get the full measure of worth out of the food consumed. The sufferer from chronic dyspepsia and the various forms of indigestion is actually as thin as a rail." Because stoutness, thus, was partly the result of good digestion that old proverb could be turned around to say, "grow fat and you will laugh" as it was not easy to be jolly with indigestion, heartburn, and other similar ills. A good cushion of fat was said to be a great preventer of the common cold and a great aid in keeping the body at an even temperature during the sometimes dramatic changes in the weather. Since the body was kept on such an even keel by its fat that induced contentment and made laughter easy. When the writer of the piece asked if laughter would make a thin person fat his answer was "Undoubtedly." Since few people breathed deeply enough it meant a large section of the lung was not only unused but was filled with stale air. "But the man who laughs heartily and often need have less fear: he clears out his lungs, he uses their full extent," he concluded.[31]

3

Oddities, Sports, Clubs, Employment, 1880–1919

In October 1881, the *New York Times* published a satirical editorial on fat women who appeared on public display in the dime museums all over America (the "freaks" in the freak shows). According to the piece, "There are always seven Fat women simultaneously on exhibition in the United States. Some of them are attached to traveling shows and some of them are exhibited in the so-called museums of our large cities, but their aggregate number is always the same. Each one is invariably described as 'the American Fat Woman,' thus implying that there is only one of the species in existence." Continuing on, the editor remarked that it was strange that it had never occurred to any scientific person to notice the fact that a private Fat Woman was absolutely unknown. "There are, of course, women in private life of great breadth and weight, but no one ever saw a real Fat Woman outside of a museum or a circus."[1]

A brief 1883 item noted the death of the "fattest woman in the world," a member of Nathan's Cleveland Circus, who apparently smothered to death in her bed. Miss Conley weighed 497 pounds.[2]

Later that same year a reporter with the *Washington Post* talked to a showman hunting talent who came to Washington from New York City to look over the fat people to be found in the dime museums in the nation's capital. The visitor said, "You may not believe it, but fat people are in great demand. The dime show 'fakes' have a lease on 'em, it appears, and the few real ones as is now on the turf have to be gobbled up by strategy for the tenting season." When the reporter asked him what he meant by real ones the visitor went on to explain he meant ones that were fat from natural causes and not manufactured. Reportedly someone wishing to obtain a fat person for a museum or circus could place an order for one, with a specified weight range, and receive delivery in 36 hours. There was said to be a doctor in New Jersey who created them by blowing them up. "The doctor came from Germany. His method is to put a pipe into the arm of a lean woman and put some kind of gas into it," explained the visitor. "The doctor found out by applying this treatment to various parts of a woman's body she could be bloated out to most any size, but son, she don't weigh any more. Sometimes when a big ballet is on in New York this same doctor is sent for to blow up the legs of the dancers." Of course, the story was bizarre nonsense, but presented straight and as though it were true by the *Washington Post*. Attempts were made in this period to "manufacture" fat people but it was done crudely by trying to add padding and skin-like coverings to an average-weight person. Such methods did not work very well and helped contribute to the fading away of the public fascination and interest in seeing fat people on public display.[3]

A news report from 1887 observed that the fall of the year was the time when freaks made a beeline for New York City — to try and get work in the dime museums after being on the road over the summer with a traveling circus or some such outfit. It was said to be worth it to the freaks since they could not earn $1 a day in any other capacity in the world. However, fat people were not especially well paid among the freaks, they averaged about $30 a week, although a tiny number got as high as $500 a week. Glass eaters earned about $20 a week; India rubber men (contortionists, double-jointed) got $100; hairy boys from Burma got $100; snake charmers $60; iron-jawed men (eaters of nails, steel, and so on) $15 to $20 per week. Highest paid freak was said to have been Jo Jo the Russian dog-faced boy, who was at one time paid $1,000 a week.[4]

Spectacle was added to the freak show when a wedding took place on the stage at Austin Stone's Dime Museum in Boston on February 19, 1889, when Alice Hogaboom (23, of Vermont) married Albert Thompson (23, of New York). Alice weighed 650 pounds; Albert tipped the scales at 90 pounds. Bridesmaid was Hannah Battersby, who weighed 810 pounds and was billed as the biggest woman in the world. In the background, immediately behind the bride and groom, were seated five women whose aggregate weight exceeded 3,000 pounds. Albert came from a wealthy family in New York that stood high in society and first met Alice in a dime museum in Manhattan when she was exhibiting her obesity for $30 a week. His family was very much opposed to the match and had disowned Albert. After he first met her in New York, Albert followed Alice around the country, courting her in season and out. The reporter joked it could not have been love at first sight for Albert "because he couldn't possibly have seen all there is of Alice the first time he looked at her."[5]

The weights listed above for the obese people were almost certainly exaggerated. That is true for virtually all of the weights given in this book for the grossly obese, say over 400 pounds, especially if they put themselves on display. It was in the interest of all the showmen of the era to lie about the weight of their fat people in the hope that the higher the weight, the greater the patronage and resultant income. It was in their interest to lie and they did. The much mentioned — and legendary fat man — Daniel Lambert supposedly weighed over 700 pounds. Most likely it was very much less.

When a *New York Times* editorial in 1905 mentioned giants (the very tall) in show business, it moved on to discuss fat people in the same business, saying, "It used to be the case that the fat man of the show divided popular attention with the giant on the same platform with him..." But then confidence in fat people had been shaken by the discovery that many of the fat people on stage were fakes. That is, often the apparent bulk was not real but merely the inflation of an India rubber costume, made up to any girth desired. Reportedly, the device was not only used for show purposes but was also employed by advertising doctors having anti-obesity mixtures to sell. Cited was a case in France where a man admitted in court he had been a professional fat man for a patent medicine man and had worn just such a suit. "Such a revelation as this not only shakes public faith in the anti-fat remedies so advertised, but it also discredits the pretensions of the fat man of the shows, making of him merely a pneumatic fantasy and hallucination," declared the editor.[6]

According to dime museum operator George A. Middleton, in 1911, "A fat woman always pays. What I mean is that she pays to have as an attraction in a side-show." Middleton was said to have been the originator of the dime museums on the Bowery in New York. He was so successful there that he branched out in many cities of the United States, having for a while a large circuit similar to the vaudeville circuits of 1911. That is, he rotated his attractions and freaks through his museums, a week here, a week there. Added Middleton, "people love to see anything abnormal in another man or woman and that is why we always featured our fat women, had then hauled in trucks, pulled by four horses, lifted with derricks and pulled off other wonderful advertising features. After treatment of this kind the fat ladies became as skittish as prima donnas when it came to salary. They had to have their raise, their special compartments while traveling, the finest hotels or they would quit." Middleton started in the business with P. T. Barnum. He had charge of concessions and, among other things, had to look after the sideshow features. During one winter's off season, while the show was lying idle, he decided to put some of his most valuable sideshow features — including fat people — into a then untried dime museum. In two weeks that Bowery place was one of the most talked about entertainment venues in New York. But, "The moving picture theaters killed the museum business to a large extent," said Middleton.[7]

Among the odd inventions was an 1884 device that was described as a sort of combined roller skate and spring engine designed exclusively for fat men. It consisted of a set of small wheels to be attached to each foot. Those wheels were combined with a spring in such a way as to be set in motion whenever a weight pressed upon them — a step, the more weight, the more speed. On ordinary roads it was estimated a man weighing 150 pounds could attain a speed of six miles per hour; one weighing 200 pounds, 10 miles per hour; one weighing 300 pounds, 25 miles per hour. As for men weighing less than 100 pounds, the new invention was thought to be of little use to them.[8]

A long article about the Holmes' Star Theater, in 1890, then being constructed in Brooklyn, called it the safest and most substantial building of its kind in America. The main entrance door was 28 feet high and 17 feet wide. "But fat people, too, will have abundant reason for special gratefulness toward Manager Holmes," explained the account. "The seventh or eighth row of seats, from one side of the house to the other, in the lower or orchestra floor, will be chairs forty-two inches wide. The ordinary seats are about twenty inches wide. The wide seats will be for fat people. Mr. Holmes says that at his former theater he usually had a number of women and men who could not sit in his seats without undergoing a great deal of discomfort, and some who could not use the seats at all, but had to be given places in the private boxes."[9]

At Lille, France in 1898 the Correctional Court had a case before it when a fat man named Payelle, a chemist, paid for a third-class ticket but because of his size he could not get into either a third- or second-class compartment. He therefore took a seat in a first-class vehicle and refused to pay the difference in the fares. In court he argued that when the company sold him a third-class ticket it put the onus on itself to find him a place in a third-class carriage and, as he could not fit into one he was entitled to take a place in the only carriage with a doorway large enough to admit him. France's Correctional Court disagreed with Payelle's arguments and upheld the contention of the railroad company, which argued that if he could not physically get into a third-class carriage he should buy a ticket entitling him to ride in a compartment of the class into which he could squeeze himself. Therefore, the court ordered him to pay the difference in the fares and all the costs of the legal action.[10]

The idea of placing a special tax on fat people was seriously considered in Sweden in 1903, but never implemented. Advocates of such a tax argued that when a man was above a certain weight he was well-fed and consequently in a prosperous condition, "and so in a position to contribute easily to the public funds."[11]

Forty fat men called on Chicago mayor-elect Fred Busse (also a fat man) in 1907 and discussed with him the possibility of organizing a Fat Men's Club with the mayor as president; it was to be a dining and political club. Busse said he was willing to join such a group but he declined its leadership. One of those 40 men, ex-senator Thomas J. Dawson (262 pounds) declared, "I miss my guess if Mr. Busse don't make the best mayor Chicago has ever had. Take a fat man and he feels so good and joyful with himself and all the world that he just can't keep from doing the right thing at all times." Another of the men, ex-senator William E. Mason (admitted to a weight of over 240 pounds but would not state the exact figure) said, "Mr. Busse's election is a complete vindication of fat men. I am in favor of a law which will prevent any man who does not weigh more than 200 pounds from holding any public office. In the coming administration we fat men will get justice. Heretofore we have been laughed at and derided. Now the next man who laughs will be sat on by the Mayor and I guess that will hold him a while."[12]

According to the lead sentence in a 1908 article that originally appeared in the *Baltimore Sun,* "This is a great year for fat men." More generally, the writer stated, "Good nature increases in men generally in proportion to their avoirdupois. You can tell by looking at a lean and hungry Cassius that he has a mean disposition. People who spend their time attending to other people's business are usually thin, and the reformer is the creature of the hatchet face and hollow cheeks." Continuing on, the piece added, "The fat man is never a fanatic, and is seldom an anarchist. He looks upon the world with kindly eyes and finds it good from its governments to its beefsteaks. It feeds him well, it clothes him well, and though he feels it has crowded a little too much flesh on his bones, he can puff and bear it." That year of 1908 was described as special for fat men because both the Democratic and Republican parties had candidates running for president — Bryan and Taft — "with big bodies, big brains, and big hearts." And, he noted, "The big man smiles with satisfaction when he opens the morning paper and looks upon their pictures. He feels that they are members of his fraternity, one in sympathy and soul with him." Of Bryan and Taft, it was concluded, "the very look of the candidates shows a massiveness and solidity that are impressive. This is a big country and it seems to call for a big President; and when the big man looks on the prospective nominees he feels that the country is safe if it chooses a man like himself."[13]

Few oddities matched the bizarre nature of a brief article that appeared in 1908 in the *Oakland Tribune.* It outlined the terribly low wages paid in Paris, France, to female workers in the French garment industry, as low as 30 cents for a day of 15 or so hours. Mentioned was a factory where women made feather boas and "The making of the boas has the disadvantage of inducing phenomenal obesity. The women so employed will become enormously fat and the doctors imagine that it must be owing to some powder or dust in the feathers." No other details were given.[14]

For the first time since it came into existence, the Public Service Commission of New York came to the aid of fat people when it investigated a 1908 report that there were inadequate stairways at the Christopher Street station of an elevated rail line in New York City. Commissioner Eustis learned from testimony given at a hearing by transit inspector Frank Bennett that much congestion existed on the downtown side of the station with the "practical stoppage" of traffic on the stairway when two fat men going in opposite directions met on the stairs.[15]

The whole situation came to the attention of the Public Service Commission as a complaint presented by the Fat People's Association. That complaint was in the form of a protest that the elevated roads' stairways were too small. Bennett testified, "The stairways are a little narrow, that is, when two persons of the size of Mr. (William Howard) Taft attempt to pass each other." Eustis then asked the inspector what would happen if Taft going up the stairs should happen to meet himself coming down the same stairs. To which Bennett began his reply, "If an irresistible force meets an immovable..." Eustis stopped him there and said the Public Service Commission would investigate further and if necessary the stairways would be widened.[16]

Nineteen-eleven saw the marriage in Dover, New Hampshire of Samuel Chesley Drew, the "pride" of the New England Fat Men's Association (456 pounds) and the former Rose Lavigne (278 pounds). When they returned home from their honeymoon as there was no carriage in the town capable of transporting the couple, they were conveyed from the train to their home on a hay truck. Drew was the head chef at the New Hampshire State Hospital and Poor Farm while Rose was also employed there, as chief nurse in the insane ward.[17]

The Irish Relief Fund Bazaar opened in Madison Square Garden on October 14, 1916, and drew a crowd of 3,000 people on the first day, it was partly sponsored by Irishmen and partly by Germans. On the ground floor were booths where people could buy various items while in the basement sideshows were featured. One of those attractions was "the world's fattest woman," or a customer could go into a canvas-enclosed area wherein was being held "The International Fat Ladies' Bicycle Riding Contest."[18]

In the field of sports and athletic events, the fat men's baseball club of Brooklyn journeyed by train to Flushing, Long Island, in October 1885 to play the fat men's team of Flushing. According to the colorful prose of a reporter, "The individual masses of rotund corpulency made up the famous Fat Men's baseball nine of Brooklyn, and they had gone down with all the speed they were capable of to test the agility of a similar set of linear and latitudinal giants from Flushing." The Brooklyn nine weighed a total of 2,211 pounds (246 pounds on average) with the biggest being a Mr. Jones at 325 pounds, who joked, "It costs me 50 cents every time I play a game of ball — 25 cents to a small boy to put my uniform on and another quarter to get him to take it off. No one was allowed to be a member of the Brooklyn team unless he weighed at least 212 pounds. "Second base was covered by a colossus whose biceps and calves of burly girth and broad expanse of shoulders displayed a wall of flesh in that strategic center," said the reporter. "The short stop was a portly Alderman, who revealed by his playing that some sinewy muscles were concealed beneath his adipose development. A full-blown Dickens's fat boy rested indolently on third base. Across the [out]field three fleshy columns had been placed for ornament, and they revealed a conscious dignity in never deigning to chase the ball."[19]

A dozen years later a fat men's baseball game was played in a city park in San Diego with all of the players being prominent business and professional men. Heaviest player was W. J. Davis at 295 pounds, a member of the Board of Public Works.[20]

Bill Reid was the new head coach of the Harvard University football team in the spring of 1905 and he declared at that time that the coming season's squad would not be called a "team of fat men." To that end he already had the players working out in gyms, and so on, to reduce their girths. Commented a reporter, "This move is without a precedent in Harvard's history, for although football demands more of its men than any other game, little or no preliminary training has been considered necessary."[21]

When the Roman Catholics of Los Angeles held their annual summer picnic in August 1897 some 3,000 people attended. As usual at such affairs baby contests took the limelight and many were held — by age category such as infants under one, babies over one and under two. Also, many track and field events were held, including a 100-yard "running race carrying baby." The fat men's 100-yard race was open to men over 225 pounds.[22]

Venice, California, was the site in August 1906 for a gathering of some 5,000 members (and friends) of the Fraternal Brotherhood for their annual seaside outing. Attendees came from all over Southern California. Among the events were the usual baby contests, track and field competitions, and a race for fat men, won by George Hood of Los Angeles.[23]

When the New York Patrolmen's Beneficial Association had opening day of its annual games, on August 7, 1906, it was reported, "The most interesting event on the programme was the fat man's race for policemen weighing over 225 pounds. Five men competed, whose combined weight was 1,350 pounds [an average of 270 pounds], all of whom were weighed in before the race."[24]

More than 2,000 people of French origin in the Los Angeles area gathered on July 14, 1911, to celebrate Bastille Day. Athletic events of various types were featured, one of which was a fat man's race, which the French called "course des hommes gras."[25]

A couple of weeks later the annual picnic of the Southern California Maccabees was held at Venice, California with a crowd in excess of 1,000 people. Featured were the usual baby contests and track and field events. Included in the latter were a 100-yard dash for men weighing 175 pounds and over and a 50-yard dash for women weighing 175 pounds and over. A fat woman's race was unusual.[26]

One month after that the Indiana Society of Southern California held its annual picnic in Los Angeles, with a crowd estimated in excess of 2,000 people. Prizes were given to the prettiest baby, the oldest woman in attendance (86), and the oldest man (81). A prize awarded to the fattest baby went to Raymond Gillman aged 20 months (35 pounds) and the prize given to the fattest woman went to Mrs. S. T. McCann, although her weight was not reported.[27]

Track and field events were held on August 15, 1913, at Washington Park in Los Angeles, but the name of the sponsoring organization was not given. Said a reporter, "The fat man's race...was the feature of yesterday's field events at Washington Park. Never before has so much adipose tissue coagulated on a single runway. Just how these inflated parties managed to get on the programme is something of a mystery. However, it is darkly hinted that they paid well for the purpose."[28]

New York's Fat Men's Association continued on as one of the more prominent and well known of such groups. At an August 1884 annual clambake gathering of the group — Philetus Dorion was president of the society — a journalist reverently declared, "Mr. Dorion is huge, he is ponderous, his obesity borders on the infinite; and the most hardened lean man cannot gaze upon his magnificent proportions without unconsciously made purer and holier." Some of the clambake crowd came on streetcars and, it was noted, "Fat men sat on each side of the street cars, and so beautiful was their development that the conductors had no room to walk between the rows to collect fares, and in some cases the watch chains of fat men sitting opposite each other became entangled or their vest buttons dovetailed." At noon the display of fat men at the gathering spot was "awe-inspiring. There was not a man among them who could catch sight of his watch chain; scarcely one who could observe his feet without the assistance of a pier glass, and none who did not weigh a fraction of a ton." Prominent among the members was Charles Wolfe (429 pounds), Peter Murphy (425 — club treasurer and secretary), ex-president Charles Bradley (he weighed 350 and 370 pounds, respectively, in the years 1871 and 1872 when he was club president, and 401 pounds in 1884). Another half a dozen club members weighed above 319 pounds and were listed in the news account by name and by weight. An official weighing-in onsite at the clambake, just before and just after eating, revealed how much weight some of the club members gained from that single meal. Philetus Dorion's weight moved from 340 to 348 while that of Mrs. Oscar Church went from 357.5 to 367.5 pounds. Most male members of the group gained from five to eight pounds each with most female attendees gaining between three and six pounds. Some past presidents and their weight in office included Willard Perkins (540 pounds in 1882) and John Fiske (358 in 1869).[29]

In Washington, D. C., that city's Fat Men's Club held its third annual picnic excursion to River View in the summer of 1893. Three steamers were chartered for the event and made seven trips, transporting 6,200 people. Sporting events included a baseball game between fat men and lean men, and a three-legged race in which only men of 200 pounds and over were allowed to participate. Several other races and similar events were held for fat men.[30]

Later in 1893, also in Washington, D. C., the first annual parade of the Jolly Fat Men's Club took place on August 31. Over half of the 200 members of the club turned out and passed along the main streets of the city — they rode in carriages; they did not walk. Notables in the group were George Mountcastle (419 pounds) and Dr. Greenlaw (385).[31]

A fight broke out in Washington, D. C., in 1894 between two fat men's clubs, both of which had scheduled their annual picnic for the same day, July 9. Both events were to include athletic events, baseball games, brass bands, and so on. The members and guests of the Jolly Fat Men's Club, "the originals," planned their event for Bethesda Park while the Fat

Men's Beneficial Association had planned a steamboat excursion to River View. Visiting fat men from such places as Baltimore, Philadelphia, and Richmond were expected by each group. The dispute started early in 1894 when a number of South Washington members of the Jolly Fat Men undertook to have inserted in the group's constitution a beneficiary (insurance) clause. Heated debate followed but the idea was voted down. Then, at a later meeting when not many of the South Washington members were present some one proposed a by-law that members in favor of a beneficiary scheme be dropped from the club. So the 50 or so South Washington men withdrew and promptly organized the Fat Men's Beneficial Association, which quickly grew to around 100 members.[32]

An 1897 article declared that there were about 5,000 clubs in existence in the United States and that nearly 100 of those were of the "eccentric order." Falling into that latter category were the One-legged Club of St. Louis, with membership open to men who had lost one leg (22 members); the Anti-Matrimony Club was a group of young women who had sworn not to marry; and the Suicide Club of Bridgeport, Connecticut — seven of the group's members had died by their own hand during the previous five years. Also placed in the eccentric category was the Fat Men's Club of Milwaukee, having 24 members with an average weight of 250 pounds.[33]

Fat men's races were an integral part of police department annual summer outings, perhaps more than with other groups and received regular mention in the newspaper. For example, a New York Police Department picnic held in June 1882 featured a huge number of track and field events, and various other athletic contests. One was the fat men's race for policemen weighing between 200 and 220 pounds. The nine contestants ran a distance of 220 yards with first prize being a china tea set; second prize $10; third prize was a family electric battery. Winner was Officer Dusher of the 10th Precinct who covered the distance in 34.5 seconds. A second fat man's race was run for contestants weighing over 220 pounds. Officer Lewis of the 25th Precinct won the first prize — an easy chair — after winning the race in 39 seconds.[34]

About 1,200 traffic officers took part in the seventh annual field day in 1915 of the Traffic Squad Benevolent Association in New York City — they were part of the New York City Police Department. There was, of course, a fat man's race, won by Officer Pat McDonald (250 pounds), guardian of traffic at Times Square.[35]

The Fat Men's Beneficial Association in Washington, D. C., had its clubrooms in 1894 on the second floor of 363 M Street, the lower portion of which was occupied as a saloon by William Wells. In July of 1894 the club was raided on a Sunday by the police after they received a tip that the bar was being run on Sundays (an illegal act). Police posted on a stakeout outside the premises watched three officers of their force (all in uniform and all on duty) being admitted to the premises after knocking on the door. Officers on stakeout then forced their way in and went upstairs to the Fat Men's club rooms where they found a keg of beer on tap, and many men drinking — including the three on-duty cops. Additionally, they found five other policemen (none in uniform and none on duty) in the place drinking beer. Charges were preferred against all the police officers found in the premises.[36]

A few days after the raid the charged officers appeared before a police trial board, for their internal hearing. A newspaper account had a subhead stating, "Testimony of five fat policemen before the trial board about the recent raid." At that hearing the three cops on duty and in uniform received a favorable ruling from the police trial board and all charges against them were dropped when their version of the story was accepted. According to those three, they had been informed by a citizen that illegal beer sales were taking place and they had gone to investigate. Admitting they had tried to run out of the premises when the stakeout team broke in, they explained they were not trying to escape but had perceived that a raid was in progress and were trying to run outside to the front of the place to head off any person trying to escape. The five off-duty cops were charged before the trial board with being in a place where the liquor law was being violated and with refusing to assist their superior officer (one of the stakeout team) when he was assaulted by the club's bouncer. All five were members of the Fat Men's Beneficial Association.[37]

While those five stood guilty before the police board for being in a place where liquor was sold on a Sunday, the charges were dismissed on technical grounds. However, the hearing was expanded into a more wide-ranging inquiry and five weeks after the raid the Board of Commissioners of the District of Columbia summarily dismissed 10 members of the Metropolitan police force (seven of the 10 were members of the Fat Men's Beneficial Association and were dismissed precisely for that connection — including the five from the raid) and, in so doing, addressed a letter to

Superintendent Moore, setting forth the reasons for their action and putting on record their ideas of what the police force of the nation's capital should be. Seven were dismissed specifically for their connection with the Fat Men's Association, one for intoxication, one for being asleep at his post, and one for impeaching a fellow officer's testimony. According to the Commissioners' letter the Fat Men's Association "was composed of policemen, saloon-keepers, and others, the policemen and saloon-keepers constituting the active members." That association had 36 members. The letter went on to castigate all the members of the club as having organized a social drinking club in the interests of the saloon-keepers and that when the officers joined the club they deliberately betrayed the public trust reposed in them and became the active tools and agents of men whose purpose was to violate the law. Such violations of the law were particularly egregious since the officers were all veterans and were thoroughly familiar with all aspects of the liquor law. A reporter observed that on the rolls of another fat men's club in Washington "appear the names of a number of other policemen." He speculated that a number of resignations from that and similar organizations would be sent in without delay. It was also said the action of the Board of Commissioners was a slap at the Police Board for the lenient and cavalier way it had dealt with charges brought against officers stemming from the raid.[38]

When the raid was not quite 3.5 years old it was reported that the fifth of the former Fat Men's Beneficial Association seven officers to be dismissed in the wake of the raid had been reinstated to the force. Only two remained off the force and one of those dismissed men was then the recipient of lobbying efforts on his behalf and was expected to be soon reinstated.[39]

For decades there had been a multitude of reports about fat men's races being held as part of police annual outings and games' days. Seemingly the idea that fat policemen might not be in the best interest of the general public to "serve and protect" was never mentioned in print. There was no mocking, satire, or irony in the reports of fat policemen's races, for example; such items were always reported straight. But police corruption in general in the late 1800s — not just by or about fat cops — had caught up with the police departments and municipal government employers in general. Rules were imposed, in the form of public service commissions, and a no obesity rule found its way into some civic employment. For the first time being obese could officially bar a person from a job.

One 1906 news report from Colorado noted that applicants for positions on the police force had to be younger and taller than in the past as, on April 6 of that year, the civil service commission adopted new rules that made 30 years the maximum age and 5'8" the minimum height, one inch taller than formerly. Additionally, "There is also a general rule against obesity."[40]

Two years later, in 1908, Willard Garrison wrote an article in praise of the civil service commission of Chicago with its standardized tests for prospective policemen and firemen, and for the commission's medical and physical examinations. An applicant for a position as a police officer had to be between 5'8" and 6'5" in height and weigh between 150 and 250 pounds. "Obesity, muscular weakness and poor physique are insurmountable barriers to the man with a craving for a place among the finest," said Garrison. Those tests were used to establish standing eligibility lists from which successful candidates were hired as vacancies occurred. Height and weight standards for the Chicago Police Department were as follows: 5'8" (150 pounds minimum, 190 pounds maximum); 5'9" (155, 195); 5'10" (160, 200); 5'11" (165, 205); 6'0" (170, 215); 6'1" (175, 220); 6'2" (180, 230); 6'3" (185, 235); 6'4" (190, 240); 6'5" (195, 250).[41]

In June 1910 legal papers were served on Theodore Bingham, former police commissioner of New York in a suit for $100,000 in damages brought against him by Captain William H. Hodgins, described as the "fattest captain" in the police department. Hodgins was once retired from the police force for "obesity" but when he demonstrated to a jury that he could hop, skip and jump like an athlete, he was immediately reinstated. However, his 1910 complaint was not about fatness. Rather, Hodgins charged in his complaint, that when he came up for promotion to the rank of inspector Bingham certified to the civil service board "maliciously and untruthfully" that Hodgins was not qualified to command because he was "stupid."[42]

General William Shafter of the United States Army who weighed around 400 pounds announced, in 1906 from retirement, that he had a profound aversion for fat men, either as enlisted men or officers. "They're no account for soldiering," he complained. "They pant, they wheeze, they snort, they choke, they grunt, they groan, they waddle, they slough through the world. Not a particle of good on earth, fat soldiers — would not have one of 'em around if I could help it." When another officer pointed out to Shafter that he was not exactly slight himself, the general replied, "Slight? No! Hell no. I've been a fat, blobby old nuisance ever since the day I tipped the beam at over 200 pounds, and right then I ought to have been court-martialed and cashiered for outrageous and malicious adiposity, sir — for scandalous corpulence to the prejudice of military discipline."[43]

Five years later, in 1915, the French military (with World War I underway) took action with respect to the so-called "cent kilos," the 220 pound and up men who had been up to that time exempt from military duty. Starting then such men were likely to be called upon for service in the auxiliary corps. French officials were then working on a law to revise all exemptions from military service. Men weighing 220 pounds and over were not considered fit for service in zones of operation but it was maintained that they were perfectly capable of guarding lines of communication and doing other service in the auxiliary department that would relieve men capable of doing the actual fighting.[44]

Late in 1907 the Philadelphia *Record* newspaper said employment agents in that city declared it was almost impossible to obtain a job for fat men because "they are regarded as beings as undesirable in industries as are the gray-haired. The employers are said to hold that the fat man is indolent. The hustler, the fast, nervous, energetic worker is sinewy, rather than fat, and does 30 per cent more work than the soft, fat fellow." An editorial in the *Los Angeles Times* argued against that position citing U. S. presidents as an example. Some thirty different presidential elections were said to have been held since the nation was formed and perhaps a score of different men had held that office — from George Washington to Theodore Roosevelt. Admitting the best of the lot (Lincoln) was decidedly lean, the editor declared, "But count the rest of them, from Washington to Roosevelt, and while perhaps few of them were soft and flabby, most of them were certainly rotund, with plenty of good adipose tissue." Also cited was one of the front-runners for the upcoming 1908 presidential election. William Howard Taft (then secretary of war) weighed about 330 pounds.[45]

Also in 1908, fat men in the United Kingdom, it seemed, would no longer be eligible to become officers in the London Fire Brigade, because two men in that department had just been denied promotion on account of their bulk. One of those had been in the brigade for 17 years and supported a wife and six children. For the prior three years he had been receiving about $9.75 weekly as a probationary sub-officer. But he was suddenly returned to the rank and file with a reduction in his salary of about $1 a week. That man's measurements were; waist 38 inches, chest 42.5 inches, height 5'7.5" and weight 179 pounds.[46]

On very rare occasions, though, being fat was sometimes the only way to get a job. On the last day of February 1909, what was described by a reporter as "more than 45,000 pounds of fat women" gathered at the stage entrance of the Majestic Theatre in New York City for a 3:00 P.M. stage call in response to an ad that had been put in the paper by the theatrical manager of *The Three Twins* company for chorus girls weighing 200 pounds and up. A line began to form before 2:00 P.M. There was so much pushing and shoving to get close to the door the lone policeman on the post found it necessary to call for aid from a nearby station. When all were finally admitted to the venue they were directed to take seats in the orchestra section while they waited their turn to audition. "There were but few, however, who could get between the rows of seats, and still fewer who could force themselves into the orchestra chairs," said the journalist. Some 200 women showed up for the audition with the three chosen for the openings weighing 385, 230, and 290 pounds.[47]

Early in 1916 the New York Civil Service Commission had just adopted rules eliding many fat men from civic jobs and was swamped with inquiries as to when mass firings would begin. One of the Civil Service examiners was asked in what departments obesity was most prevalent. He replied that it was to be found in every department, adding, "There is one mass of abounding girth in a department who has a record for exterminating swivel chairs. He weighs about 250 pounds." New obesity rules were a function of the job grouping categories. In group I, which included indoor workers, it was permissible for the jobholders to be moderately stout. That class included clerks, bench artisans and professional men and jobs in that category did not call for vigorous muscular development or sustained effort. Jobs in Group II required a moderate degree of physical ability such as would enable the incumbent to perform continued outdoor labor or to walk long distances and carry small loads. Jobholders there were entitled to bear even less fat. In Groups III and IV were included people who performed severe manual labor, and firemen and policemen. Jobholders there were supposed to have no fat on them at all.[48]

In order to protect the pension system as well as to insure efficient service, the municipal Civil Service Commission of New York City imposed a sweeping set of standards in 1916 on those who applied through it for civil service jobs in New York City. Disqualifying defects, from any and all consideration for employment, were such items as chronic alcoholism, drug addiction, cancer, tuberculosis, and "extreme obesity," defined as "Excessive obesity is a condition where the least possible horizontal circumference of the abdomen is greater than the greatest possible horizontal circumference of the chest."[49]

4

Causes and Cures,
1880–1919

Put forward as a cause of obesity in 1883 was the general idea that women grew fat more quickly than men, possibly on account of their sedentary lives, although men, when inclined to fatness, attained a much larger growth. Up to about the age of 40, unless fatness was hereditary, and provided that a proper amount of exercise such as walking, horseback riding, running or rowing was indulged in, both men and women, but especially men, retained a rather natural corpulence, went the theory. When women reached the age of 40, however, and especially so with those "who have fulfilled their duty toward the world" (that is, given birth), they assumed what was termed in French embonpoint, which, literally translated, meant fine condition. However, declared the article, "Fatness come in what shape it will, cannot fail but prove a discomfort, accompanied as it always is, with slowness of movement, shortness of breath, sleepiness, palpitations of the heart, and proneness to apoplexy and sudden death."[1]

The question as to whether water was fattening or otherwise was one that was much discussed with ordinary tap water regularly blamed as the cause of human obesity, by people in the medical and scientific communities. Prior to the mid 1880s it was generally asserted that the victims of obesity should mortify the flesh and reduce the fat by abstaining as much as possible from liquids and remaining in a continual state of thirst. Then, around 1885, the "hot water cure" became fashionable with the consumption of hot water supposedly causing a weight loss, provided always the water was taken as hot as possible, "painfully hot and in great quantities." Experiments made in Paris in 1886 by Dr. Debove contradicted both of those ideas and should have put water into its proper place, with respect to human obesity. His controlled experiments indicated that, provided the same amount of solid food was consumed, large or negligible quantities of water made a man neither thinner nor fatter. Despite Debove's finding a reporter commented, "Still, it is quite possible that the old theory of thirst cure and the new theory of hot water cure may both be correct." However, he acknowledged that both of those conditions violated the natural conditions of health. And that left him to conclude that perhaps the oldest prescription, "Keep your mouth shut and your eyes open" when followed with judicious limitations was the best. "Eat less, sleep less and walk more are safe injunctions, provided they are obeyed in moderation."[2]

While Debove's work should have settled the issue of water as a cause of obesity it did not, at least not right away. Investigations by Dr. Lorenzer of Erlangen, Germany, purported to show that the increasing or decreasing of the quantity of liquids in the diet had a corresponding effect on the accumulation of fat. Lorenzer advised people troubled by obesity to restrict the amount of fluids used, remarking, "Thin persons seldom drink much." Debove's results applied only to water and not to any other fluids. But at this time fluids were all too often lumped together and treated the same way. Water was the same as beer, which was the same as coffee, which was the same as wine, and so on. No allowance was made for the sometimes vastly different caloric values of different fluids.[3]

A French biologist named M. Levan proposed the theory in 1888 that obesity was a nervous disorder, to be treated by the avoidance of mental and physical fatigue with a diet of eggs, soup, milk, rice and potatoes.[4]

Later that same year an article that originally appeared in a publication for women called *Dress*, told of a secret for women troubled with obesity, "namely that bodies exposed constantly to the sun gain such activity of the blood forces as to prevent any excessive forming of adipose matter." Readers were warned, though, not to suppose that, on the other hand, plenty of sunlight was conducive to leanness. "Not so, for the really healthful condition is neither fat nor lean, but shapely and plump, and the sun's rays quicken the nutrient functions, producing a beautiful and elastic roundness of form."[5]

Still in 1888, the idea of inherited obesity was raised. It was stated in a news account that the obesity of the Queen of England "has been bequeathed to all her feminine descendants. It is difficult for the average American to reconcile royalty with fat, but it must be done...It is rather odd that none of them inherit the Prince Consort's trim figure." Various princesses were then cited as evidence of the theory with the author concluding it was not a particularly gracious thing to do, his dwelling on the physical characteristics of Queen Victoria's feminine descendants, "but the facts are impressive to sight-seers. It destroys all the charm and romance of royalty, in spite of the most vivid imagination, this remarkable tendency to obesity in the Victorian era."[6]

An article that appeared originally in the *Chicago Record* in 1896 asked itself the following question in print, "Why is it that nine tenths of the women in public life are more than 36 inches around the waist?" Rather than produce a specific answer to his question the author of the piece offered some general thoughts. He argued the female wasp-waist (so attractive to men) was brought about only through fetters, processes against natural growth, and so on. And that such women remained psychologically curbed and fettered by social conventions beyond the aspect of clothing; that is, they were not assertive. "But the assertive woman, the woman who has broken away from the fetters and is leading the beleaguered hosts of emancipated femininity in a headlong assault upon the ramparts behind which the tyrant man is entrenched in fancied security is the woman of goodly girth and muscular frame," he concluded. "Her disregard of the mandates of fashion is as great as her contempt for masculine admiration is scornful."[7]

W. R. C. Latson was a medical doctor who edited *Health Culture Magazine* (New York) in 1903. After declaring that perhaps few conditions were more misunderstood than obesity he noted, "People say 'fat and healthy' as if the terms were logically associated. Few seem to appreciate the fact that obesity is a disease — that the fat person is never well, and that in many cases he is in a dangerous condition." Obesity he defined as the result of the formation of an excess of low-grade tissue, which, owing to a deficiency of the eliminating organs, was not removed from the body, as it should be. As to causes, that formation of tissue was due to one or more of the following: a) the taking of food in excess of the digestive powers; b) incomplete digestion resulting from too frequent eating; c) the taking of any fluid or solid substance that alters or interferes with the digestive process (such as candy, tea, coffee, alcohol, pastry); d) the taking of an undue amount of fluids with food (causing digestive juices to be diluted and thus unable to convert the food mass); and e) general constitutional inactivity, the result of which is insufficiency of secretion of digestive fluids. According to Latson fat people could be divided into several classes; some were strong, some were weak; some had soft mushy tissue, while the tissue of others was firm and solid. Furthermore, the location of the fat deposit varied considerably as the adipose tissue was usually deposited in those portions of the body where there was the least motion. For example, said Latson, the woman who carried herself well but who sat a great deal, would find the fat settling around the hips and thighs. Why did the fat not settle around the abdomen in such women, he mused? His answer was because the mere act of standing erect meant active work for the muscles of the abdomen and prevented the accumulation of adipose in that region. On the other hand, the man who stood incorrectly — as 99 percent were said to do — allowed the abdominal muscles to remain flaccid, resulting in very little activity in that region and so the fat settled there." Left unexplained by Latson was why virtually all men stood incorrectly while almost all women apparently did not.[8]

A minor stir was created in New York in 1903 when an author named Bronson Howard declared that women of wealth and position in New York (the elite 400) drank too much for their own good. One who commented on the issue was Dr. Watson Savage, head of the Savage physical culture institution — every winter its clients included many of the cream of New York society struggling to maintain their looks, and so on. With respect to his female clients, Savage said it was not true that such women were drinking more and that none had ever come to his facility because they needed treatment for the results of excessive drinking. "Possibly obesity, of which some women come to be cured, might be called the result of too much drinking," he added. "But the cases of obesity I have treated during the past few years have not been of that kind." All women then wanted to be slight, explained Savage, and they were willing to give up a great deal for that. "They know that nothing will fatten them more quickly than alcohol. Now people know as they never did before what the result of their imprudence will be. Women realize that cocktails and champagne will puff them up." Savage declared it was then inexcusable to be fat because so many women had shown that it was possible to avoid that condition by healthy exercise and diet. "Women, therefore, who think of their appearance are more careful about drinking than they ever were. And the women who have social position and obligations are more careful than any others to avoid the kind of a life that is going to bring them to the state they are trying so hard to shun. For their appearance and for their health they are drinking less than ever."[9]

Over a decade later, in 1915, a piece that appeared originally in the United Mine Workers' *Journal* stated, "Not all hard drinkers are fat, but the tendency of alcoholics to obesity is too marked to escape notice. A well-known doctor says it is because the alcohol usurps the function of the fat, which accumulates." According to that doctor, "It is noticeable that those addicted to the use of alcoholic beverages often reveal a tendency to corpulence which is proportional to their use of the drug. The fatness is not a sign of health. It is not even an indication that alcohol is harmless. It is merely the result of the complete oxidization of the substance of alcohol by the human body." Under this theory the body would oxidize a two-ounce quantity of alcohol in 24 hours and would do it so completely that no trace of alcohol could be found in any excretory substance. That meant the unnatural heat produced in the body by the presence of the stimulant answered, at least for the time being, for what would otherwise be produced by the expenditure of fats and carbohydrates. Those latter items were the fuel stored up by the body and normally burned up in the production of necessary bodily heat, and that expenditure was avoided. The fat was therefore stored up in the body unused and corpulence was the necessary result. "This, of course, is not a normal condition nor a proper process. It becomes more unnatural with the increasing use of alcohol," warned the physician.[10]

Writing editorially in *American Medicine* (Philadelphia) in 1907, a physician expressed the view that in experimenting for the elimination of poisons in the body that "may cause obesity," scientists had ignored the factor of nervous disorders. That cause, he asserted, "is most noticeable in the obesity of childhood, but is equally evident in that of adults. They are defective in many ways, lacking in vitality, rarely living to old age, subject to complaints of nervous origin, and prone to certain infections." If the idea was raised, said the editor, that a man was fat because he ate too much then it was necessary to ask why the man ate too much. In the opinion of the editor, "The fierce, swinelike appetite is of itself a stigma of abnormality, and though there is some evidence that cases exist in which the food ingested is not excessive, it is quite evident that it is too much for the work done." With the adult obese, as Rabelais was cited as having observed, "appetite comes with eating," which caused a journalist to conclude, "The more the patient eats, the more he wants to eat. It is this ravenous desire that our expert [the physician] ascribes, in some instances to nervous causes."[11]

A London, England, physician, who counted among his patients many well-known London women, pointed out in 1910 the effect of too much automobile riding on the figure. He declared, "At the risk of making myself unpopular I have had to forbid motoring to several of my patients who have consulted me regarding their growing embonpoint. Those who have followed my advice have succeeded in regaining their figures." And, "Motoring surpasses in luxury any form of locomotion yet invented. The seats are so tilted that one is forced to lean back among the cushions at such an angle that all the muscles are relaxed." If all that wasn't bad enough, said the medical man, "Add to this the exhilaration which rapid movement produces and the increase of appetite engendered by plenty of fresh air, and you will see that motoring contains most of the elements which make for adiposity."[12]

A woman's columnist (on beauty hints and the like) named Lina Cavalieri had her column appear regularly in the *Washington Post* in the pre–World War I era. Her regularly occurring by-line read as follows; "By Mme. Lina Cavalieri, the most famous living beauty." In her column of October 8, 1911, she wrote, "The fear of fat is constantly before women, and I am glad that it is so, for what we fear we try to avoid. There is no dissenting voice among the nations, Turkey excepted, that fat is a burden to the body and a destroyer of grace." She said the study of the problem was bringing new facts to the surface about the causes of fat and the treatment of fat. "For instance, a professor in the Paris Academy of Medicine has concluded that fat is not a disease, but a symptom of disease. It proves, he says, that there is a derangement of some function. Perhaps the kidneys are not doing their work well. Perhaps the liver is unusually lazy. Perhaps the digestion is faulty." Cavalieri granted they were interesting theories with perhaps a grain of truth in each one of them since they all came from "unquestioned authority." But one of the latest theories was of the most practical value to women, she thought. "That is the conclusion that the cause of superfluous flesh in the woman of 30 and the cause of superflu-ous flesh in women of 40 is different. In other words 'thirty fat' and 'forty fat' are of different origin, and being of different origin are of different kind and cure." Within this theory the cause of obesity in the 30-year-old women was due to one of three factors; "suralimentation," which was merely indigestion, improper distribution of food elements in persons of rheumatic tendency; latent dyspepsia; or pre-existing nervousness. For the older women the obesity was due usually to "nervous trouble."[13]

Famed superstar actor Lillian Russell was listed as the author of an advice article on how to keep from getting fat, published in 1913. Com-menting that some people ate very little and yet still got fat, Russell explained, "this tendency is hereditary. More than half the fat people are fat because the character runs in the family." She also commented on other factors, saying, "Age has a great influence. People seldom become unduly fat before the age of 40. And sex also has something to do with the mat-ter for women are far more frequently fat than men."[14]

Physician Dr. R. R. Daniels authored a 1914 article that explained the cause of obesity. In his view the fat of the body always came from a single source, the food and "Regardless of whether the fat man may be a light eater or a heavy eater, he always eats and digests more food than his body uses up. Nature, in her economy, saves this excess by storing it in the form of fat." While he had that part right he drifted off into fantasy, "While an excess of any food may be converted into fat in the body the sweets and the starches, such as breads of any kind, cereals and potatoes, are the usual sources of fat. It is of these things that the fat man always eats more than he needs." Foods that made fat were "force-producing" foods under normal conditions, he explained, but as the body got into the habit of converting these foods into fat the individual lost vigor. Further, too much fat overworked the heart, overstrained the arteries and tended to bring on degeneration of the kidneys. An early death from worn-out organs was said to be the fate of the average fat man. As well, the obese had a diminished disease-resisting power with typhoid fever and pneu-monia being particularly fatal among fat people. For Daniels, the only rational method to cure obesity was to, first, reduce the amount of "force food" to just what could be used in the body and, second, to get the body into the habit of using up more food, and out of the lazy habit of converting the food into fat. That meant the fat person should eat a sufficiently small amount of starchy foods to permit a constant reduction in weight until it was down to normal and "that he should get plenty of fresh air night and day, wear light clothing, especially underwear, take a daily sponge bath, and follow systematic exercise."[15]

A 1914 article that appeared in the *Washington Post* warned of the danger of excessive potato eating. According to the author of the piece potato eating had become a habit not because potatoes contained enough nourishment to carry on life, but because they were cheap, easy to prepare and bulky enough to fill up the stomach. The potato consisted almost entirely of starch and though that had a place in the diet, warned the writer; it was not capable of building up strength and muscle. He concluded, "Excessive use brings an inevitable trail of anemia, obesity and auto-intoxication."[16]

Susanna Cocroft, a self-styled women's beauty consultant, contemplated the causes of obesity, in 1914, and declared, it "is due to a combination of luxurious living with a lack of some definite, animating purpose. There are so many women who are sitting down even when they are standing up. Their figures show the same lassitude, the same limpness of muscle, exhibited by a tired person leaning back in a low, deep soft chair. The person who stands or walks in this fashion cannot have the curves or lines of the perfect figure. The first thing she needs is a bracing interest in life." Cocroft also stated, "mature women, especially if they are well to do, eat too much for the small amount of exercise that they take. If they would do more work the food they consume wouldn't injure them. Often I tell my rich women patients in Chicago to scrub their own floors. The modern dances are also good exercise."[17]

By late in this period, though, the medical establishment had largely reached agreement on the cause of obesity; the quackery and silliness did not disappear but was limited mostly to the quacks. Dr. Walter B. Bloor of the department of biological chemistry at Harvard University Medical School gave a 1917 lecture on "Fat" at that institution. To the disappointment of many of those in attendance, reportedly, he did not give expression to some new theory concerning the reduction of obesity. Admitting obesity was undesirable, Bloor said, in his lecture, "The principal cause of obesity is overfeeding. Unfortunately persons approaching middle age do not know that they are overfeeding themselves. As less exercise is taken, less food should be eaten. Persons who worry require more food than persons whose minds are at ease, for worry results in greater physical, heart and mental action.[18]

Dr. George Van Ness Dearborn of Cambridge, Massachusetts, argued, also in 1917, that obesity came down to energy level; it was a matter of intake versus expenditure. As long as they were in balance everything was well but if intake exceeded expenditure then fatness resulted. It did not matter how much the intake was — high for a lumberjack, medium for a clerical employee, or low for a bed-ridden person — so long as a balance was maintained. Dearborn negated the long-standing nonsense that certain foods were bad, that is, fattening. Still, Dearborn said some people were born fat; others achieved fatness, while still others had fatness thrust upon them. With those who are "born fat," argued Dearborn, "our immediate interests can have no quarrel; rather must we quarrel with these unfortunates' forebears. Pathological obesity undoubtedly looks more and more as if it were due to some still unknown defect in the metabolic apparatus." He remarked that if had recently been shown that unusual smallness of the lungs (thus minimizing the destruction of fat) was another factor in the tendency to obesity. By adequate systematic exercise of the proper kind the lungs may readily be much enlarged and accumulation of fat be prevented or lessened, sometimes to any desired degree. However, Dearborn did argue, "The great and culpable majority of the obese achieve their uncomplimentary fatness. These people, or most of them, are quite needlessly unhappy because their lives are inefficient, and if they persist, as needlessly short-lived." In Dearborn's view the most important way in which to reduce one's dietary intake was to use the continuous will power of restraint, "very few of really fat people have sufficient will-power, however, month after month to reduce the diet in a systematic and scientific manner." With respect to those who had fatness thrust upon them, or as Dearborn called them, "the adipose victims of circumstances," he explained, "some of these are, of necessity, engaged in oversedentary occupations; some are helpless cripples; some are ignorant; some are indifferent — i.e., of swinish disposition; some are wise but weak-willed; and some are strong-willed enough, but foolish or perhaps indifferent to the length of life or to the full measure of physical and moral manhood or womanhood." Concluded the doctor, "But with this, although a considerable class of the obese, we need not here concern ourselves, for the scientific conditions are like unto those of the persons who achieve fatness — although, humanly speaking, far harder, because less often relieved."[19]

Cures advanced ranged from the sensible to the bizarre, from well-intentioned scientists to unscrupulous quacks out only to lighten wallets. At the Fourth Congress of German physicians, held in 1885, the first subject discussed was corpulence. Ebstein advanced the opinion that drugs were of little service in reducing the amount of fat "and that an entire change in the regimen — including both change of diet and of manner of living — was necessary." Any method, said Ebstein, that reduced the general nutrition, and thus removed fat, was a failure: the fat alone had to be removed. The method employed must not require the individual to give up his business during treatment, else it would not be generally applicable. Also, the method used must be capable of being continued indefinitely without producing unpleasant results, because individuals predisposed to corpulence by heredity or constitution must keep up the diet for a long time. One method, continued Ebstein, was to cut off all fatty foods. But because carbohydrates could be changed into fat in the body, that was not reasonable. The object was to prevent the formation of fat in the body and "To secure this it is necessary to regulate the proportion of albuminous, starchy and fatty foods, so that perfect nutrition shall be secured, but no excess fat produced. The necessary amount of fat for a healthy man is 142 grains (a grain equaled .002286 ounces, .0648 grams) per diem," explained Ebstein. If that amount was reduced by 50 percent, a part of the amount necessary for nutrition will be taken from the body to compensate for the reduced allowance in the food, and thus the excess of fat may be removed. "Under this system the individual does not suffer the distress which is felt by those who are cut off from all fatty food, and the results are more successful and agreeable than those of the Banting system," Ebstein added. "In the Banting system the diet is chiefly nitrogenous, which often causes indigestion." Within his system, Ebstein gave nitrogenous food, with a reduced allowance of starch and fat, in sufficient quantity to keep up the general nutrition and working strength, but not in such amounts as to overload and embarrass the organs that digested proteins. Also, "the necessity of muscular exercise of sufficient force to produce free perspiration is insisted upon" in his system. As to the conference in general, it was reported "all agreed that the use of medicine for reducing corpulence was to be avoided."[20]

An example of a bizarre cure for obesity could be seen in a craze that swept America and the UK in the last few years of the 19th century. According to an article that appeared originally in the New York *World* in 1896, corpulence was a subject constantly brought up in the offices of physicians. Hardly a day passed without the query being heard, "Oh, doctor, what shall I do? I am growing so stout?" In reply to the oft-repeated questions one doctor replied "Carlsbad" (a spa), another said "ride a wheel" (bicycle), while a third suggested some nauseous compound, or perhaps starvation. And, remarked the reporter, "Day after day elaborate accounts of new treatments for obesity are detailed in both medical and lay journals. Some of these are not without their good points, while others are positively dangerous. At all events, the great majority of the 'cures' require such an amount of persistence and self-denial that the cases in which they prove beneficial are not very numerous. Massage and various movements, when performed in a systematic manner have always been highly rated in the treatment of obesity. Sweden (where massage and the movement cures originated) had been the home of the 'cures' for many years." Then the journalist told of the latest remedy for corpulence, a remedy apparently first reported in the *London Graphic*, a cure described as simplicity itself, which "requires in the main that the sufferer shall turn somersaults; how many and how often the *Graphic* report does not say." One danger pointed out associated with this new treatment was appendicitis, with the new treatment playing an important, but unspecified, role in the production of appendicitis. Several observers had called attention to the fact that people who indulged in gymnastic exercises (often involving somersaults) such as trapeze work, and so on, "are particularly liable to the disease mentioned." Concluded the American reporter, "May not one hope that as a result of this treatment uncommonly stout people of prominence will no longer be characterized as fat? It is well known that fat persons, men and women, are always eager to reduce their flesh. Fancy Mr. Cleveland, Mr. Reed, Gen. Harrison and other eminent persons being attracted by this newest and latest remedy for excessive embonpoint and putting it into practice."[21]

Two years later, in 1898, a Cynthiana, Kentucky, man arrived home for supper one night and found his wife on her head with it wedged between the bed and the wall in such a way she could not move. When finally extricated the woman swore she would never again try turning somersaults to reduce her fatness. She had sent $2 to a New York mail order firm for a cure for obesity. In return, she received a leaflet explaining the somersault cure.[22]

That fad was still on the go in 1902. At that time an account in the *Los Angeles Times* reported the latest London, England novelty was the somersault cure for fat women. A West End physician's house had been fitted up as a luxurious gymnasium where aristocratic patients turned "somersaults on Swedish principles," in the hope of reducing their obesity. According to the account the "cure" was said to be "most efficacious."[23]

Home steam bath cabinets were also often touted as the cure for fatness. A full-page ad for such a device in 1899 in the *Los Angeles Times* hailed it as being able to cure nervous troubles and debility, clear the skin, purify the blood, cure rheumatism, "women's troubles," la grippe, sleeplessness, obesity, neuralgia, headaches, gout, sciatica, piles, dropsy, blood and skin diseases, liver and kidney troubles, and more. That Vapor Bath Cabinet could be had for $5, and for an additional $1 the buyer received the optional "head steaming attachment."[24]

During the summer of 1899, Dr. William T. Cathell of Baltimore declared he had discovered a simple and sure cure for fatness. Overweight people began by drinking a big glass of Kissingen water (mineral water) 20 or 30 minutes after breakfast, another at the same interval after the noonday meal, and another at the same interval after the evening meal. On the next day the person did the same thing exactly, except substituting Vichy water for Kissingen. The next day it was back to Kissingen, then back to Vichy and so on from day to day, always drinking the water in the same way. Said Cathell, "If any healthy person weighing less than 300 pounds, with simple uncomplicated overfatness, will persistently continue to take them thus, week after week, he will gradually lose fat until he comes down to medium weight and stoutness, and be correspondingly relieved of the discomforts and the dangers of obesity; after which their use should be discontinued." If at the end of the first two weeks of treatment the patient was not at least four pounds lighter, Cathell advised the patient to add a few teaspoonfuls of lemon juice to each glass of Kissingen, and one teaspoonful of aromatic spirits of ammonia to each glass of Vichy. He also advised the consumption of "acidulous" food and drink on the Kissingen days, and an avoidance of them on the Vichy days. It was also reported that in the wake of such attention, the demand for

Kissingen and Vichy in Baltimore "has become tremendous." Dr. Cathell added that after a patient was cured of fatness he must not overeat at meals and he also admonished patients to be "very temperate" in the use of fatty and oily food, sugary or starchy food, and in the use of alcohol. "If you do not heed these admonitions, you may fat up again," he warned. Also included in the article was an "incomplete" list of cures achieved from following this regimen. A fat grocer reduced from 310 to 239 pounds in 11 weeks; a barkeeper from 223 to 180 in 19 weeks; a lawyer from 191 to 173 in 14 weeks; a real estate agent from 173 to 151 in 12 weeks; a clergyman down 16 pounds in nine weeks; a 28-year-old woman down from 286 to 264 in 13 weeks; an actress from 173 to 166 in seven weeks; a young woman from 149 to 143 in five weeks; a bus conductor from 183 to 174 in six weeks; and a 41-year-old woman from 173 to 160 in 11 weeks.[25]

Some eight months later an article remarked that moderation in diet had long been recommended to reduce weight but never more so than then, and especially so in conjunction with certain mineral waters, the use of which was said to be strongly advised by medical authorities. For instance, the *British Medical Journal* went so far as to say the efficiency of Apenta, a Hungarian aperient water, "for the systematic treatment of obesity is clinically established" while a leading Berlin medical journal "says that Apenta produces a reduction of fat in the body without detriment, as the general health of the patient suffers in no wise, the cure running its course in a satisfactory manner."[26]

Then there was the posture cure, part illusion and part something else. According to a 1901 story, "The apparent size of the abdomen may be made less by a correct standing and sitting position. A lounging position, which lets the body fall in a heap at the waist line, relaxes the muscles and favors a fatty deposit just where it is most detrimental to the beauty of contour of a woman's figure." If the abdominal muscles were not permitted to become relaxed, but were held firmly in position by an effort of will, "there will be an apparent reduction in flesh about the hips and abdomen before even a single pound is taken off." Readers were also advised to do abdominal exercises each night and to use a straight-front, comfortably-fitting corset, which "reduces the apparent size of the figure. Tight lacing is a grievous error. Billows of fat overflowing above and below a constricted waist never tend to diminish the size. Exaggerated curves serve only to render obesity more prominent. The more evenly distributed the excess of fat, the less it attracts notice." Lastly, additional advice was that massage rollers and a pint of hot water formed a "powerful and harmless anti-fat combination. Vichy and seltzer are also excellent to drink in place of water to quench thirst."[27]

Closely related to the posture cure was the 1902 stooping remedy. Christine Terhune Herrick was the author of cookbooks and a proponent of, or perhaps deviser of, the stooping cure. She declared, "Few women who have any inclination to flesh take kindly to the exercise that forces them to bend over or to stoop. Yet this distaste, if indulged in, is likely to increase the very trouble they deprecate." Herrick then told the story of a fat man who had led a sedentary life operating a tobacco store. To cure obesity, his doctor told him to give up his shop and to engage in the selling of small mechanical toys on the sidewalk (such sidewalk vending was common at the time). That involved, of course, a lot of bending and stooping. In a few months he was said to have achieved "astonishing results" in reducing his size. "It is in line with this that physicians recommend stooping and bending exercises to patients inclined to too much embonpoint," explained Herrick. "As women go on in years they are prone to accumulate flesh about the abdomen, and such exercises as stooping, to wipe or brush the floor or to pick up this and that, is distinctly beneficial." Making beds was also described as good exercise to reduce fat, as it involved mattress turning.[28]

According to a piece that appeared originally in the Philadelphia *Record* in 1902 a physician looked with disgust at a diner wherein most of the customers were fat. Taking in all the pendulous paunches and double chins in a sneering glace the medical man wondered, "Why will men and women be disfigured with corpulence when the remedy is so simple and sure?" And that remedy was the "natural one" that would occur to an animal or a savage — fasting. "Let the fat man or the fat woman fast a week, two weeks, three weeks, or a month — fast till he or she be thin enough — about once a year, say, and corpulence, that most unsightly and unhealthy condition, would vanish from the face of the earth," was the solution in the article. In conclusion, the article asserted, "Fasting would be a very good thing for fat people to do regularly. They would then keep always shapely. During their abstinence they would live on and consume their own fat as hibernating animals do."[29]

Typical of the array of quack remedies for obesity was an ad that appeared in the *Washington Post* in 1904 and promised the reader a free trial offer of "Obesity Food" by return mail for sending in his name and address and no money, to Prof. F. J. Kellogg, 171 Kellogg Building, Battle Creek, Michigan. It was a standard ad of the era with text extolling the virtues of the product and the usual testimonial. According to the ad text, "Excess fat is a disease. It is caused by imperfect assimilation of food. Nutriment which should go into muscle, sinew, bone, brain and nerve does not go there, but piles up in the form of superfluous fat, which clogs the human machinery and compresses the vital organs of the body, and endangers health and life." However, pitched the ad, Obesity Food, taken at meal time, compelled perfect assimilation of the food and sent the food nutriment where it belonged. And, "It requires no dietary or starvation process. You can eat all you want. It makes muscle, bone, sinew, nerve and brain tissue out of excess fat, and quickly reduces your weight to normal. It takes off the big stomach and relieves the compressed condition and enables the heart to act freely and the lungs to expand naturally, and the kidneys and liver to perform their functions in a natural manner...No dieting, exercise, or exertion is necessary." That product pitch used the same come-ons that made quack remedies big sellers then, a century earlier, and right up to the present time. The buyer was promised something for nothing, weight reduction through the use of the product with no need to diet, or exercise, or change eating or living patterns at all. The obese person who had spent one or more years gaining 50 or so excess pounds but did not want to make any alterations in his life, or make any exertion or effort to reduce, was always ready, and remains so, to purchase such a nostrum.[30]

Even the United States government had a cure for obesity. Through the Agriculture Department, in 1907, it was conducting experiments to show the overweight how to lose weight and the thin how to gain weight. To the fat person who wanted to lose weight, the federal government said, "Eat little, sleep little and drink less." The fat person "must not drink a drop of water or any other liquid one hour before eating nor until an hour has elapsed after he has finished. If he can make it two hours so much the better." For breakfast he was advised to have eggs, toast and coffee, or cocoa without sugar. Lunch was to be limited to a simple piece of meat or a cup of consommé or some fruit. Dinner could consist of any kind of meat, in any quantity but no vegetables other than tomatoes or cucumbers. No bread or butter was allowed. Tea could be consumed provided it contained no sugar. "The fat man to get thin can eat nothing containing starch or sugars. He must eschew such foods as peas, beans, beets, potatoes, cauliflower, cabbage, parsnips, bananas and any other class of food of the starchy or saccharine variety," explained the Agriculture Department. "He can eat any kind of meat except veal, for this is held to be fattening. He must live mainly upon oranges, apples, grapes and other acid fruits, and the three or four vegetables that tend to thin the blood. He must drink no milk and very little water. Alcoholic beverages of all sorts are barred."[31]

Madame Jacques arrived in Washington, D. C., from France in 1908 with a bunch of corsets and a proposal to introduce corsets into the U.S. Army and the U.S. Navy both to reduce weight and to cure other problems (unspecified but perhaps posture-related). A reporter doing the story treated Jacques as something of an eccentric. She also wanted to see her corsets worn by fat federal cabinet officers and by President Theodore Roosevelt. Jacques said, "President Roosevelt is such a darling. He will love blue. And won't he be a dainty specimen of manhood. Since he has lived at the White House he has become too stout. But when he has worn a corset a few weeks he will improve. Then he won't have to be so strenuous. He can lay back in his easy chair and let Secretary Loeb do all the work." She complained that the way men dressed was all a mistake. That if they wore corsets and stockings that came up above their knees they would not be "physically good-for-nothing at the age of fifty...When I get through with Secretary Taft he will be able to dance the Virginia reel, walk a tight rope or balance himself on his hands. His 300 pounds of flesh will disappear like an icicle." And with respect to military officers threatened with discharge by Roosevelt because they were out-of-shape, Jacques declared, "I guess they are now lying awake at nights worrying over their growing girths and increased waist lines."[32]

In Philadelphia at a session of the American Gynecological Society in 1908 one item discussed was the idea of curing obesity by surgery. Famed German gynecologist Dr. F. Pfannenstiel, a member of the kaiser's council, read a paper in which he pointed out the transverse incision, which he had pioneered, was the best method to apply to stout patients. A visiting surgeon from Baltimore agreed, saying he had used the transverse incision on an obese patient "and taken out more fat than he could hold in both hands."[33]

At a 1909 meeting of the Society of Internal Medicine in Paris, Dr.

Marcel Labbe read a paper on the treatment of obesity. Essentially, he believed that there was only one method of treatment, "we must decrease the alimentary income and increase the expenditure of energy." Among the foods he recommended for reduced consumption, or complete elimination from the diet, were the fats, breads, pastries, and sweets. As well he advised the use of salt should be reduced as much as possible. Labbe added, "One of the most frequent of lay methods is to stop drinking. This is an important error which may even become dangerous" because the absence of water could affect the kidneys. Also recommended was, "In reduction by means of exercise, the latter should be dosed like a medicine; walking is especially to be recommended" and "the treatment of obesity by medicine should be absolutely given up, for it is injurious."[34]

A reader wrote to a woman's household hints column that appeared in the *Los Angeles Times* in 1909, asking the columnist for information about the "standing" cure for obesity. Apparently it involved standing for 20 minutes and the reader wanted to know if it meant standing still or if one could move about, and do housework, for example. Said the columnist, "One must not take exercise that will weary the body and retard digestion. To take a long walk or to tramp up and down the veranda, as is the custom at watering places, after a hearty meal, provokes dyspepsia. The stomach needs rest in order to carry on aright the work committed to it. The same objection applies to active housework. Lounge about the room or the porches after eating, standing erect all the time, or stroll slowly about the lawn, never forgetting the erect position. You must not bend over or hurry yourself." Citing an example of the efficacy of the standing cure, the columnist told of a woman who had spent four months practicing the "standing regimen" and lost five inches of girth from her hips, three inches from her bust, and two inches from her waist.[35]

Newport, Rhode Island, was a fashionable resort area in America in 1911 and every now and again one of the Eastern newspapers in cities such as Washington, New York, Philadelphia, Boston, and so on, reported that a woman who had been a shining light in society was in bad health, had broken down under the strain of her social duties, and was sent off to a Newport resort to recuperate. According to one journalist what was not said was that often that bad health had been "caused by the use of a dangerous anti-fat drug, with which fashionable women in Europe first experimented. Women in Newport have been using this drug ever since fashion decreed that a truly fair one must be slender." Th main ingredient in many of those drugs — usually obtained from mail-order quacks — was thyroid extract, which had dangerous side effects. Said the *Journal* by the American Medical Association, "In most cases of obesity treatment by thyroid is essentially illogical and treatment by diet and exercise is the logical method. In his conclusion the journalist declared, "emphasis should be laid on the fact that in almost every case the obesity is due simply to over-eating or to lack of exercise or to a combination of these."[36]

Journalist Ada Lee published a lengthy interview in April 1912 in the *Washington Post* with a well-known dispenser of quack obesity remedies of the day, Marjorie Hamilton Cunningham. On the surface it looked like any other celebrity interview conducted by a by-lined reporter. However, the piece was so uncritical, so fawning, and so egregiously worshipful that it likely was a planted piece. Probably Hamilton, or her media staff, wrote it and paid directly or indirectly for its insertion in the newspaper. "I have just met and talked to a real woman. When instructed to interview Marjorie Hamilton, who has won fame and fortune by teaching fat people how to grow slim by her drugless treatment, I didn't know just what kind of a person I expected to meet," enthused Lee. "A slim, exquisite, girlish young creature, radiant with health and youthful beauty and with the most beautiful skin I have ever seen, came toward me with a genuine sure-fire smile beaming at me across her outstretched hand." Hamilton told Lee that it was her proudest boast that the best advertising she got was not what she paid for in the newspapers and magazines but the "free and unsolicited testimonials" given by those whom she had reduced to the slimness of desire. "That is why I have succeeded where others have failed. I have really relieved people of their burdens of fat, and I have done it without drugs, without tearing the bodies of delicate women to pieces with strenuous and injurious exercises and without starving them," she explained.[37]

Hamilton's story was that she had been a calendar model, had led an indolent life and was eventually dropped as a model because she became too fat. She then tried literally dozens of fat reducing remedies but none of them worked. "Then I tried exercises. I was always fond of sports and outdoor games, but the dreary monotony of these exercises grew every day more trying as I followed out the courses laid down by the physical torture experts until every bone in my poor little body ached, and I decided even fat was better," she elaborated. "I tried starving myself, but the result, while it took pounds off fast enough, left me hollow-cheeked and dim-eyed, and I felt my vitality slipping away from me." Reduced to desperation she came upon a newspaper account of a domestic tragedy that became a moving factor in her life. Marjorie read of a wife who killed herself because her husband had ceased to love her after she had become fat. "The thought that I, too, some day might fall in love with some man whose heart would remain closed to me because my ungainly, ugly fat body robbed me of that attractiveness that all men desire in the woman of their hearts, chilled me. I went to work to solve the problem of how to regain my slimness," she said. She studied all sorts of things, conducted various experiments, and so on, and finally found the cure for obesity. Deciding to let "the world share my secret," Marjorie scraped up the money for her first advertisement, wherein she told her story, "That I had reduced myself at the rate of a pound a day after the other so-called cures had failed; that my treatment was drugless; that it did not entail a starvation diet, and that it did not require back-breaking and body-racking exercises."[38]

Hamilton explained that the astute public, which could winnow the chaff from the wheat of every advertised proposition, was with her. Marjorie increased dramatically her advertising expenditure and enlarged her office facilities. "I found then, as now, that society women and actresses were my best customers. This word of mouth, this whispered name from fat woman to fat woman has been my best friend and my greatest advertiser." But she quickly said her patrons were not women only and that thousands of men owed their regained health and a reasonable waist-line to her. Her clients were said to include men famous in business, in politics, in the church, and in the professions, "It is not always vanity that prompts them to take my treatment but more often the desire to be rid of an incubus of flesh that worries and annoys them." Reporter Lee marveled at length about Hamilton, about her building a fortune from nothing, and so on. "I would have quit a thousand times if my own personal interests alone were at stake, but I felt that I owed my sisters a duty," said Hamilton. "I felt as though this knowledge I have received had been given to me as a sacred trust for the benefit of humanity. My necessity had made it profitable to me, but I should like to be able to benefit all those who suffer from obesity." She claimed to have given her publication, "Fat Reduction Without Drugs," free to tens of thousands of people who had written to her asking for it. Lee echoed Hamilton's sentiments when she said, of her interview subject, "She feels that she is performing a duty to humanity." Hamilton was interviewed by Lee at corporate headquarters in Denver where "hundreds of women" assisted Hamilton in sending out free brochures, and so on. With regard to exactly what type of cure it was that Hamilton had for obesity (including cost, method, length of treatment, and so forth), not a word was said. Inquiring reporter Lee had, apparently, not bothered to inquire.[39]

Less than two months after that so-called interview was published, Marjorie Hamilton Cunningham and her husband Walter C. Cunningham, described as "beauty doctors" and advertisers of an obesity cure, were indicted by a Federal Grand Jury, in Denver on June 6, 1912, on a charge of fraudulently using the mails. Evidence against them was obtained by Post Office Inspectors in Denver and Washington, D. C. More than a score of witnesses were summoned before the jury, from all over the nation, to bring charges against the Marjorie Hamilton Company — mainly women who wanted to reduce their weight. It was alleged the defendants sent out 2,500 letters a day across American advertising their obesity cure for $15. If the prospective patient was not responsive to the first letter then others followed, each decreasing the price of the cure.[40]

The Hamilton case dragged on for over a year before it reached a jury. In Denver on June 25, 1913, Judge Lewis ruled that the efficacy of the treatment was not an issue in the case, and neither was the fact that money was not returned when demanded. A prospectus for the Marjorie Hamilton firm said, "and having perfected this plan — I have come to the conclusion that mine is the same method that was used in ancient times by those beauties who held the power of nations in their hands. In my search for the simple method which I offer you, I read of Cleopatra, of the Empress Josephine, of Helen of Troy and of all the queens of beauty of ancient times, and I feel sure that my method, which has been perfected, must have been the same used by those beauties of history."[41]

After a two-week trial in Denver the Hamilton case went to the jury on Monday, June 30, 1913. After taking some 100 ballots, and deliberating for 54 hours, the jury failed to reach a verdict, standing at seven to five in favor of conviction before being dismissed by the judge.[42]

During 1912 a story spread that a new remedy was available — tapeworm pills for curing fatness. Supposedly the pills contained the heads and first links of tapeworms, with food enough to keep the worms' heads alive for a week. Surgeon General Blue of the U.S. public health service (to whom a query was directed), Dr. Anderson, director of the U.S. hygienic laboratory, and Dr. Doolittle, acting chief of the U.S. bureau of chemistry, all stepped forward to say they had never heard of any tapeworm pills and that such things were impossible anyway.[43]

Yet two years later, in 1914, discovery by U.S. officials that tapeworms were being sold in capsules as a cure for obesity was said to have caused the promoter to flee Cincinnati. Investigation of the many anti-fat treatments on the market was begun by the federal food and drug bureau several months earlier.[44]

Lina Cavalieri returned with a column at the start of 1913 that contained one of the more bizarre remedies for fatness. First, she pointed out the drawbacks of exercising for women trying to reduce; "to be beautifully feminine a woman must suggest softness, as does the cat. Overexercise causes the muscles to bourgeon and harden, as the blacksmith's muscles do, and may give the curiously set and hardened expression to the face so unbecoming to women. Women were not made for hard, continuous tasks of any sort." Then she detailed the method of a "clever corsetiere" (unnamed) whose reduction method was said to have melted away the fat from a score of Lina's American friends as if by magic. At night before retiring the method required the obese person to drop a Turkish towel into boiling water, wring it out quickly, and place it about the hips and abdomen. As soon as the towel cooled it was to be removed and the process repeated. That was to be done six times in a row and the result was the same as if the person had steamed his face. That is, the pores were then wide open and were to be "fed" with a reduction lotion or cream. And the formula the corsetiere believed in was as follows: alcohol, one quart; camphor gum, two ounces. That solution was to be made up and then rubbed vigorously into the hips and abdomen. Camphor was called the active reduction agent and, explained, Cavalieri, "It does its work so quickly that in a week I have known women to lose five pounds through its use."[45]

A 1913 news story remarked that the usual remedy for obesity was "under-feeding or muscular exercise, and either may have bad effects on the enfeebled condition of many fat persons." To solve that problem, said the account, French experiments had shown that electric stimulation could provide automatic exercise for the muscles, without producing any fatigue.

Dr. Nagel-Schmidt, a German physician, had built a specially designed apparatus for applying such treatment to the obese. The device consisted of a wooden reclining chair with 10 electrodes (two for the patient's back, two for the seat, two for the calves, two for the abdomen, and two for the thighs or chest) through which passed an electric current. According to the report, "The electric treatment has the same effect in reducing flesh as ordinary muscular exercise, with no harmful consequences."[46]

Some eight months later, in 1914, Professor Bergonie of Bordeaux, France, according to the British medical journal, *The Lancet*, was said to have invented an electric bed in which the passage of the current through the body of the subject set up organic combustions similar to those brought on by muscular exercise and led to the reduction of obesity. As part of his work Bergonie studied the energy of the organism and thus noted the periods when the energy required for digestion was at its greatest. He discovered that the least suitable hours for meals were between noon and 1 P.M. and between 7 P.M. and 8 P.M., precisely the hours during which most Europeans ate. Meal hours for a "rational" system, said Bergonie, would be as follows; principal meal of the day at 7:30 A.M.; a second meal of 300 to 400 calories taken at 4 P.M.; finally, a third meal of 700 to 800 calories consumed at 8:30 P.M. or 9 P.M.[47]

A German physician (unnamed) had made a special study of adiposity and its cure and in 1913 came out with the following declaration, "Fat people ought to wear as little clothing as possible. In fact, they ought to wear no clothing for as much of the time as conditions will allow." He argued that fat was in itself a disease when it became adiposity but that every person should be "plump," being defined as having fat in certain parts of the body, and having a layer of fat of no great thickness that underlay the skin for its protection. For this medical man the taking on of too much fat was evidence of the faulty assimilation of food. Therefore, too much was being made into fat and too little into the harder tissue of the muscles. It was for that reason, he continued, that many medical people insisted their stout patients take all the exercise they could, "for exercising serves the double purpose of correcting the malassimilaiton of food and burning up the fat already accumulated by the action of the muscles. Fat is, so to say, 'burned up' by exercise, the little globules being melted away by the heat of the activity of the muscles." If it were possible to oxidize the fat in our tissues, he added, it would melt away just as it does when put into a frying pan, but exercise was indulged in by the overweight only at a great expenditure of will power. Under the no clothing theory a fat person should wear as little clothing as possible so the oxygen of the air could act upon the fat through the pores of the skin, "for while oxidation is not as rapid in this way as it is by the muscles, it is more continuous and does take place, as is plain from the hardened fat of the hardy, exposed person, when compared with the flabby fat of the coddled stout man or woman who is always wrapped in heavy garments and furs." And, "Under the action of the air the fatty globules lose much of their moisture, and become hard, shrinking somewhat and serving the purpose for which nature intended the fatty layers — protection for the more delicate tissues beneath it."[48]

Platinum injections as a cure for obesity were brought to the attention of the Academy of Medicine in Paris in 1914 by Doctor Tissier. "The results obtained are slight compared with the promises of certain advertised preparations, being a maximum of 500 grammes a week, but the cure is highly acceptable to patients, as loss of time, fatiguing exercises, and alimentary privations are unnecessary," declared a reporter.[49]

Later that same year, in Vienna, Austria, it was reported that Baroness Bertha von Suttner, the Austrian writer who had devoted most of her life to the cause of peace and who was awarded the Nobel Peace Prize in 1905, had died at the age of 71. She had been ill for three weeks and the reason for her death was said to be, "She was undergoing a cure for obesity which her constitution proved unable to bear."[50]

During the summer of 1914 the drug specialists at the U.S. bureau of chemistry conducted a series of tests on the so-called fat reducing remedies then extensively advertised. As a result the department warned the public to be aware of all such preparations. According to their report, "No other class of preparations exploited to humbug the people has a wider sale, and in nearly every instance are absolutely worthless. In many cases where patients seem to lose weight this result is attained by the hot baths and exercises recommended as an accompaniment in taking the medicine." The only ways the department's specialists knew of to safely lose weight "are rigid dieting, and strenuous exercise, and those to be effective must be continued over a long period of time."[51]

5

Reducing, Diets, and Exercise, 1880–1919

An 1882 article that appeared originally in the *Boston Globe* had a reporter interview one unnamed man in Boston who had determined to lose weight. He was 5'7" tall and weighed 270 pounds. When the reporter asked him if he took any of the anti-fat remedies so common then or if he used something like the Banting system, he replied, "I discounted Banting, following a much more rigid course." Although he admitted to having eaten enough for two men at a meal, under his new regimen he limited himself to just two meals a day, at 8 A.M. and at 4 P.M. Consumption was limited to beefsteak mainly, six to eight ounces at each meal, with two ounces of bread toasted hard. Nothing else, except on occasion a change from beef to mutton, but no vegetables, no pork, and no veal. With respect to liquids he said he drank no water, except in sips: "Fleshy persons always are tempted to drink large quantities of water. Now, let them sip their water and it will quench their thirst just as well. I usually drink a cup of tea without milk or sugar." He did admit that he suffered a good deal from hunger under that regime but did find some encouragement every morning when he weighed himself, "no one can successfully diet to reduce flesh unless he weighs himself regularly." During his first month on this diet he lost 22 pounds and a few months later he had lost weight to the point that he could walk a mile or ride a horse. He smoked 15 or 20 cigars a day, explaining, "Smoking doesn't seem to be injurious to me. I had to do something to keep my nerves soothed." After an unspecified amount

71

of time on the diet his weight was down from 270 pounds to 190 pounds, and his waist size down from 58 inches to 40 inches. "According to insurance tables a man of my height and build should weigh about 158 pounds," he added. "I presume I could diet down to nearly that, but I am satisfied."[1]

According to an article that appeared first in 1882 in the *Annual of Phrenology and Health*, people, especially ladies, who came into the professional hands of such practitioners, asked what they could do to be less fat or stout, while others wanted to know how to gain weight. Admitting people could be "constitutionally" fat or thin the reporter allowed that obesity was mostly determined from living habits. "In nine cases out of ten, those who are burdened with obesity, those who have red faces and pimples, who are so fleshy that they cannot exert themselves without getting out of breath, who are too plumb to be graceful or comfortable, get into this condition by means of what they eat," said the author of the piece. In his opinion, fat red-faced people who were inclined to pimples were blondes while fat brunettes had rough complexions but no pimples or redfaces. Advice given to the overweight readers was to eat sugar very sparingly, exclude butter or oily items, and especially omit puddings and pastries that were rich with lard or butter or sugar. People who ate such items, he continued, became "loaded with fat" because those food items "tend to produce fatness and not strength or vigor. Such food provides nothing for the upbuilding of brain or muscle. It will often be found that fat people are very weak."[2]

According to an article in the *New York Times* at the start of 1884 the only method of treating obesity that had proved successful "has been that popularly known as Bantingism, but it is generally conceded that the remedy is worse than the disease." The remainder of the article was given over to satire with a discussion of the "brigand" method of weight reduction wherein the Duke of Calvino was captured in Sicily and held for 35 days before being released after his family paid a ransom demand. When kidnapped he had been very fat but upon his release he was found to be of normal weight. During his captivity, the Duke was allowed to eat nothing but bread and cheese and to drink nothing but water. Joked the article, "According to the Banting theory this diet ought to have increased the Duke's fatness" but it did not.[3]

Five months later an article in the same newspaper complained about the Banting diet, "to many patients it was so weakening that for one who has been relieved by it a dozen have experienced actual injury. It is easy to become thin by not taking sufficient food to supply the waste which is continually going on, though in this case, the cure is worse than the disease." Professor Ebstein had come along then to scorn all such "starvation remedies" offering instead, fat as a cure for obesity, such as in eating a lot of fatty meats. Banting permitted his adherents to eat any fish except salmon but Ebstein allowed all, including pate de foie gras. However, Ebstein did forbid the consumption of sugar, sweets of any kind, and potatoes in any form. Alcoholic drinks were permitted to the extent of two or three glasses of light wine at dinner, but beer was taboo.[4]

A man by the name of Professor Huxley announced in 1884 that Dr. Schweninger of Munich, Germany, had discovered a new method of reducing weight. It was never to eat and drink at the same time but to let two hours intervene between eating and drinking. Reportedly, he had cured Germany's Prince Otto Bismarck of a tendency to obesity in that way. As silly and bizarre as that method was it did have some lasting power.[5]

Six months later, in 1885, the Detroit *Lancet* described the four plans for reducing obesity: a) the eating of nothing containing starch, sugar, or fat, called the Banting system; b) the eating of fat, but not sugar or starch, called the German Banting; c) the wearing of wool and sleeping in flannel blankets (instead of sheets), or the Munich system; d) not eating and drinking at the same time, or, rather, allowing a couple of hours to intervene between eating and drinking, the Schweninger system.[6]

Near the end of 1886 an article enthused over the German's method arguing the success of Schweninger in reducing Bismarck's obesity without any injury to his health and under a regime the patient found comfortable, "has led to a reconstruction of the systems of reducing fat. Most systems have been based on the idea that fat people eat too much and particularly too much of certain kinds of food. This is true in many cases, and yet the mere abstinence from food has not been found satisfactory." That was because it had no permanent value since the person disposed to obesity had to continue to abstain from a reasonable quantity of food in order to keep down his fat. But, "Almost always, except in the case of gourmands, the result is a general weakening of the vital powers with loss of mental vigor." Very few people who were not excessive eaters were inclined to too much adipose and had injured themselves by abstemiousness to their efforts to reduce their fat, he argued.[7]

The article summarized the Schweninger method by observing the system "considers fatness a disease, not to be cured by denying a proper amount of food. The essential feature of the treatment is to do as far as possible without fluids. It regards the fluids as responsible for the condition of fat-making. It does not deny the patient a reasonable amount of wholesome food; it involves no severe self-denial in any thing except fluids, and to a minor degree in fats." Discouraged by the system was the liberal use of butter and cream and some other forms of fat although fats were not forbidden absolutely. But it did insist strongly on the least quantity of fluids; it forbade the drinking of water as far as possible. "It insists that water shall never be taken with meals; that it shall be taken only under particular conditions, and then sparingly. It regards a tablespoonful of water as an injurious quantity that is to be taken only when it is impossible to abstain any longer," said the report. Therefore, it followed that thin people could indulge in water freely with benefit, "Indeed, all systems of making people plump urge the most liberal drinking of water."[8]

Medical doctor John Wilson Gibbs outlined in 1893 his experience in treating U.S. President Grover Cleveland with the Schweninger method. At the time Gibbs wrote his article Cleveland weighed 300 pounds, 75 pounds above his normal weight and was "greatly distressed physically in consequence." Said Gibbs, "Inasmuch as I had the honor before of treating him for obesity and had succeeded in reducing his weight from 306 to 235 pounds without any deleterious consequences, it is at once assumed that I am again called upon to apply the Schweninger cure to our popular President." Confidently, Gibbs predicted Cleveland would submit immediately to that treatment and that while submitting to it he would be perfectly able to execute his presidential duties "and at its termination will be seventy-five pounds lighter, or stronger and a better man, physically, mentally and in every other way. What is more the excess of fat with which he is now afflicted will never return. That is a disease which can be easily cured." In order to explain away the obvious problem that Cleveland had previously submitted to the Schweninger method but the fat had not stayed away, Gibbs said he had no doubt Cleveland regretted he did not adhere to the treatment two years earlier until the prescribed limits of time had expired. "This time, however, I am confident he will [stay the course] as he is growing older all the time and will not care to undergo another and another treatment every two or three years," he emphasized.[9]

Gibbs declared that in every case where the system of the German professor was strictly followed the cure was enduring. He cited Bismarck as having been reduced from 246 to 186 pounds within a period of three months, some 10 years earlier, with the cure being permanent. "Now Bismarck, instead of having the appearance of a heavy, distressed old glutton, resembles an athlete in every way," said Gibbs. He is bony, strong and muscular, and walks with the erect manner and springy stride of a champion pedestrian. His complexion is clear and almost pink, while his general health is as good as it was in his younger manhood." Trying to explain what fat was Gibbs said it was the oily concrete substance deposited on the cells of the adipose membranes under the skin and in various other parts. Obesity was the accumulation of fat under the integuments, or in the abdomen, or in both situations in such an amount as to embarrass the several voluntary functions. If the obesity could not be made to disappear, warned the doctor, fatty degeneration of the heart was sure to follow. Excessive fat, like extreme emaciation, was a disease founded on some chronic disorder, generally the kidneys. "The fleshy man or woman who has passed the 200-pound limit — unless of gigantic stature — can only be regarded by the eye of science as one suffering from disease and a fit subject for the care of a physician. People should not delude themselves with the idea that it is healthy to 'laugh and grow fat' for there never was a celebrated man who was fatter than his fellows but that effect resulted from abnormal or unhealthy conditions." He cited the "gross corpulence" of Edward Gibbons (historian of the Roman Empire) and traced it back to a sickly childhood. Dr. Samuel Johnson was said to have dated his obesity from the time when he became prey to a "morbid melancholy." Allowing that excessive fat could come from the disorganized condition of some vital organ from early childhood, Gibbs admitted that more frequently it was the outgrowth of excessive indulgence in foods and liquids in more mature years, as in the case of Bismarck, and English statesman Charles James Fox. Besides the physical dangers that came from obesity, cautioned Gibbs, there were also mental dangers to consider. With an accumulation of fat came sluggishness of the vital organs and necessarily of the brain.[10]

What was the remedy for excessive fatness, wondered Gibbs. In reply to his own query he said, "A single application of the laws of nature; no sweating, no banting, no starvation, no weakening, no laborious exercise. It is the Schweninger method which I have applied to Grover Cleveland

and which will be applied to the nation's chief again." As far as Gibbs was concerned it was a matter of first discovering the cause of the obese effects and then removing the reasons for "the unnatural and unsatisfactory condition of the patient and the cure will soon follow. Once properly reduced in weight by the system a man remains so." That is, the treatment specifics under the Schweninger method varied according to the conditions in each individual case. For example, "In one the use of starch food and sugar — within certain liberal limitations — will be allowed, while in another, the hydrocarbons will be rigidly excluded from the bill of fare, at least until their permissibility is clearly indicated by certain changes in the physical conditions. The primary thing in each case is the condition of the patient's kidneys and heart." Cleveland's weight was to be brought down by diet alone, with no exercises to be done. Probable meals for Cleveland were as follows: breakfast; one cup of tea or coffee with a little milk and sugar, six ounces; three slices of stale bread; two eggs or two to three ounces of either fish or meat. Dinner; eight ounces of meat or fish; vegetables such as spinach, cabbage, string beans, asparagus, tomatoes or beet tops; four ounces of farinaceous food such as rice and hominy; liberal amounts of fruit; wine in moderation. Supper; two eggs or lean meat, six ounces; one ounce of salad or radishes; one slice of stale bread (one ounce); four ounces of fruit; white wine in moderation; malt liquors to be avoided.[11]

Gibbs went on to discuss some of the other methods of reducing then in vogue. First he declared that all Banting or "semi-starvation" systems had been proven failures, "That of Banting himself, who was an undertaker and not a physician, conspicuously so. All of his patients besides himself as they commenced eating heartily again after nearly starving to death gained back all the flesh they had lost and many pounds besides." Then he mentioned the Salisbury system then in vogue in England, a method he considered to be probably the worst of all. Under that system no breakfast was consumed but upon arising in the morning the adherent drank a pint of water, as hot as possible. Half an hour later one pound of beefsteak, chopped as fine as possible, was eaten, after the outside had been warmed over a fire and the inside left quite raw. A little bit of stale bread was eaten with the meat. At half past two in the afternoon another pint of hot water was taken. And that was it for the day with nothing more consumed until the next morning's hot water. Fat was quickly shed under Salisbury, admitted Gibbs, but as soon as the patient quit the regime he regained all the weight he had lost, and more. Nor could anything be gained by excessive exercise, citing boxers who lost weight while training for a fight only to gain it back quickly after the fight. Another point raised by Gibbs was, "Over indulgence in sleep is sure to bring about a diseased condition of the vital organs, and more specifically the kidneys. This of course leads to obesity." Numerous examples proved that point, he argued, citing inventor Thomas Alva Edison. He was not fat but supposedly he had demonstrated by experiment how even he could gain flesh by sleeping. In one week he slept 14 hours and in the next 22 hours. The result was a net gain of six pounds in seven days. "A fat man should never sleep over seven hours and if he reduced that number to six all the better," counseled Gibbs.[12]

A 1901 article that appeared first in the New York *Ledger* and was reprinted in the *Washington Post* showered praise on the "celebrated" German physician Schweninger, who had reduced Bismarck's weight nearly 100 pounds and who had invented the reducing system that bore his name. "It treats obesity from a different standpoint than that of diet alone. It aims to improve the condition of the heart and liver, which often have a tendency to disease in fleshy people," explained the piece. "It has no cut-and-dried rules, as in the case with most systems, but is adapted to individual conditions. In some cases sugar and farinaceous foods are allowed in moderation, while in others they are strictly prohibited." The great advantage of the Schweninger system over all the others was said to be that the weight reduction was permanent. And it was permanent because the axe had been laid at the root of the trouble and the diseased tendency to undue fat production had been fundamentally checked. In the Schweninger system, continued the article, all watery articles of diet were to be avoided as far as possible, although thin beef and mutton soups were allowed. Only six ounces of bread and farinaceous foods were permitted per day with those six ounces to consist of gluten or stale bread or dry toast. Water was allowed in moderation between meals. On the blacklist were fat soups, sauces, spices, cereals, macaroni, sweet potatoes, pastry, puddings, pies, cakes, and milk. Tea and coffee with milk could be taken. For dessert fruit was recommended, with the preference given to grapes, oranges, cherries, berries, and acid fruits. Vegetables permitted included squash, turnip, asparagus, cauliflower, onions, celery, cress, spinach, tomatoes, radishes, lettuce, and greens. Readers were advised that the Schweninger system was not one a person could self-practice but could only be under-taken under the guidance of a medical practitioner, after a thorough phys-ical examination that determined the latitude in diet allowed. That, in turn, was dependant on the condition of the vital organs. According to this piece exercise was made a factor in the reduction of flesh by this sys-tem with the patient frequently made to climb hills or ascend and descend stairs a given number of times daily to improve the action of the heart. The general health was said to be "almost invariably improved" by this method. Despite the warning the Schweninger system was to be under-taken only under the guidance of a doctor, the article concluded, "Enough hints may be gleaned from the above to enable those who are verging upon the lines of unbecoming stoutness to keep within the desired weight."[13]

The "Adonis" of the New York bar, Roscoe Conkling, was reported to be growing very fat, in 1885. His attempts to check his increasing obe-sity by athletic exercises had proved fruitless. Indian clubs, sand bags, dumb bells, walking, and rowing were all used in his unsuccessful efforts. Conkling then weighed nearly 300 pounds. Supposedly one day in May 1885 while crossing the City Hall Park he dropped a silver dollar and was detained several minutes by his vain efforts to recover it. Finally, he paid a small boy 10 cents to pick it up for him.[14]

How could obesity be reduced, mused an 1885 news account, before supplying its own answer. Recourse to starvation, anti-fats, dieting by measure and the swallowing of acids were all dismissed as not only absurd but suicidal. Then the writer of the piece attacked the Banting system for the same reasons that so many others had done in the past. "A strict reg-imen is the only cure for obesity," he thundered. "Fat is supposed to pro-duce fat. Such is not the case. Fat, combining with the carbohydrates and albuminous compounds acts directly against obesity." Fat was said to check all "nitrogenous waste" and to appease thirst as well as hunger. The main thing to do in order to correct corpulence was to abstain from eating starchy and saccharine foods. Vegetables rich in albumen, however, made desirable dishes that he recommended. Potatoes, though, were never to be eaten. Fish and all kinds of meats could be eaten at any time but beer and malt liquors were generally to be avoided, because of the carbohydrates contained therein.[15]

Fruit was discussed as a valuable article of food in 1887, with few peo-ple said to see its worth but that those who did recognize its value ate fruit every day. The article argued that a common belief that eating fruit caused diarrhea was false and that the author of the piece had spent the occasional day eating nothing but fruit and never had diarrhea or looseness of stool; on one day he ate seven pounds of strawberries. Then he mentioned the curative power of fruit — the "grape cure" then a fad in France and Germany and which supposedly was a cure for many diseases due to overeating. On the first day of the cure the patient was given one pound of grapes to eat; that amount was increased day by day until the patient could eat five or six pounds a day. At the same time the other food the patient usually consumed was gradually lessened until the diet consisted of nothing but grapes. It was a diet said to cure obesity and many other complaints. In conclusion, the reporter said that in America that cure could be carried out using strawberries, gooseberries, cherries, and plums in place of grapes.[16]

Doctor Helen Densmore proclaimed in 1889 that all women should be as slender and supple at 50 as at 25. She was described as perhaps as well known and successful as any New York specialist who had followed on the heels of Banting and attacked the problem of flesh reduction. It was said, "Corpulent and dyspeptic board of trade men and o'er plump matrons of the 400 just now sit mournfully beside the scales in her reception parlor" because Densmore was withdrawing from practice. "Men and women should not allow themselves to grow stout as they grow older," Densmore added. "It is never necessary to have too much flesh to be carried gracefully." The reporter who spoke to Densmore added that "fair, fat and 40 need not go together as adjectives" and that to greatly exceed one's normal weight was prima facie evidence of impaired nutrition. The food taken in was used in forming an undue deposit in the subcutaneous tissue. Neither the heart nor the lungs could act easily and healthily, being oppressed by the gradual gathering burden. "To run the race of life no man or woman ought to be handicapped by a weight which makes active movement difficult, upstairs ascents difficult, respiration thick and panting," he said. "Fat itself is a disease as much as emaciation, and its opposite extreme."[17]

When the journalist who spoke to Densmore wondered what started a woman piling up the "detested pounds" he speculated it could be some shock to the nervous system, childbirth, a bout of sickness, a great sorrow or grief. And if the tendency to fatness was hereditary any of those other items would be even more likely to lead to obesity. However, he did acknowledge the growing "luxurious habits in eating" had more to do with obesity than any other single cause. The habits of women, a lack of exercise, the indoor life, and so on, all fostered the problem although he thought it was a mistake to ascribe too much importance to the sedentary life, as many people did. Admittedly, the tendency to sedentary habits was much stronger in women than in men. In order to lose that extra weight the reader was advised to stop feeding herself with fat and heat-producing food. The body called for about two pounds of carbonaceous elements weekly and if the person stopped supplying them the body would be driven to absorbing the stored up fatty tissue and so destroy or burn it. That was said to be the foundation for scientific flesh reduction. Readers were advised to eat only two meals a day "but as to quantity you are not in any way limited. You must remember that all oleaginous food, as fat meat, butter, gravy, milk, nuts, and Indian corn is a direct contribution to obesity. In addition to these the hydrocarbons are elaborated in the system by potatoes, rice, tapiocas, arrowroot, beets, peas and the sugar and starch of bread." People following this advice were told they had to live on a nitrogenous diet as much as it was possible, "You want to take into your system fibrine, albumen and casine, which repair the waste of tissue and are not convertible into fat. Of course you can not eliminate the carbohydrates altogether, but you want to reduce their proportions at once and appreciably, and there will result a very perceptible change in your physical condition." To accomplish that, lean meat had to be eaten with any kind being allowed but the best and more nourishing was said to be beef. "Eat of tenderloin steak as heartily as you choose. Eat lean fish, except salmon. Eat salads. Eat vegetables to supply bulk, turnips, cabbage, any vegetables except potatoes, beets and peas. Eat any fruits. Do not eat any bread. Do not eat pastry, do not eat desserts; do not touch butter; do not touch sweets of any description. Do not eat anything in the preparation of which flour has been used. Do not drink coffee or teas," went the lengthy advice. With respect to the question of whether or not to drink water, the reporter said the taboo on water was a common fallacy, as people did not grow fat because they drank water, but they drank water because they were fat. "You can drink all the water you please," he said. "It will be better for the digestion, however, if you take it hot instead of cold." He was in favor of exercising as a good thing that promoted health but that it was not necessary to exercise to lower weight, remarking that a lazy woman, if she tried, could reduce her weight without doing any exercise at all. Nevertheless the prognosis for women who dieted properly was not good. "Less than one in five of the women who begin it will persevere ten days. They haven't the resolution. A woman who is ambitious to be healthy ought to carry it just far enough to regain her normal weight, but she won't do it. She will stop far short of that, satisfied with being a little less fat than she used to be."[18]

One of the talks at a January 1890 meeting of the New York Academy of Medicine was given by Dr. Walter Mendelson, on the "Physiological Treatment of Obesity." As a result, it was said, most of the "stout physicians" of the town assembled in Manhattan to hear the talk. He approved of reducing obesity by natural means, by reducing the albumin, the fats and starches in the food. Mendelson condemned the Banting method because "the intestines were unable in any animal save a dog to get rid of the immense accumulations of meat which that system prescribed." Concerning the fattening qualities of water Mendelson said they were "unquestionably important and that too much water was an evil which should be carefully avoided." And, he added, "Persons with heart disease had a tendency to grow stout, and the excessive use of water tended to promote heart disease, for such use increased the volume of blood, and threw upon the heart a supply which it was not able to provide for."[19]

An 1891 article in a French journal announced the discovery of a simple means of curing obesity, which was attributed to a medical officer in the French army. That method consisted in never eating more than one dish at each meal, no matter what the dish might be, "and a person may consume as much as the stomach can bear and satisfy the appetite without the least reserve. Nevertheless, nothing but the one dish should be taken; no condiments, or soups, or supplementary desserts should be allowed." According to one person who tried the diet the partaking of just one dish, be it meat, fish, or vegetable, brought on a sense of satisfaction much sooner than if a variety of dishes had been partaken of. Supposedly, it had been used successfully on many people — one being a colonel in the French army who was threatened with dismissal, as he was so heavy that it required two men to lift him into the saddle. After utilizing this method he became, it was reported, "thin in a few weeks."[20]

Writing in the *New York Times* in 1893 a journalist observed that the number of systems recommended for the reduction of fat was "infinite." An English vegetarian journal held that for people to reduce obesity by living on lean beef and water was false in principle — it was merely starvation — and although they would certainly become thinner using such a method, they would at the same time reduce their strength and bring down their constitution. On the other hand, a simple diet of brown bread and various kinds of fruits was claimed to be a far better means of reducing superfluous flesh than the use of any nostrum, and it would, moreover, invigorate the body and keep up the strength. In the view of this vegetarian journal the diet should be accompanied by proper exercise with walking being the most suitable for fat people, because the whole body was exercised through walking and not one set of muscles at the expense of another. "The general diet should be plain and simple. Rich and elaborate cookery causes persons to eat more than is good for them, and brings on undue obesity and many disorders," it concluded. The reporter went on to say that fat people always had a better time of it when they were taken ill "because, if they cannot eat for a day or two, their system is supported by their fat and they will often live through an illness that would kill a thin person." His advice for a person who found himself getting too fat was for the person to reduce his intake, to eat less at each meal, and to let himself always be hungry when the time for eating came around. "If he, further, drinks nothing between meals except the glass of water prescribed by many of the best modern practitioners, about an hour before breakfast and an hour before retiring for the night, and takes regular exercise, he ought, under normal conditions, soon to attain the proportions at which nature has decided that he shall enjoy perfect health."[21]

Shirley Dare, in the *Philadelphia Inquirer* in 1893, declared the "charred bread" diet was useful in reducing flesh and should be tried before a person spent money on quack obesity cures. Under this diet all bread eaten was coarse wheat meal bread, baked the deepest brown, not quite burned, but very hard and crisp. That bread, with acidulated tea and drinks of every sort mixed with lemon juice would, it was said, "reduce flesh, correct disorders of digestion, and leave one with a very light complexion besides." Salt water baths, free exercise, and a restricted diet could be combined with this bread and lemon cure, but all three without the coarse, hard bread and acid did much less than with them. Then the bladderwick cure was mentioned, an obesity cure that some people were making a great deal of money out of, it was the extract of a marine weed that could be found along the shore, focus vesiculosus was the scientific name. First the weed was burned then the ashes were saved, boiling water was poured over them and the concoction was drunk. Besides obesity bladderwick was rumored to also work on other complaints such as dropsy and rheumatism. In general, concluded Dare, "I hear the obesity cures don't suit all constitutions, as people find themselves gaining steadily under the treatment; but the burned bread and lemon juice is pretty sure. It is easily tried."[22]

An 1893 recommendation observed first that the most serious danger from fatness was the accumulation of fat around the heart and lungs. Readers were advised that mild aperients should be taken frequently, and also stewed fruits. All alkalines were described as valuable, and lemon juice was desirable in every form. Green salads, watercress and asparagus could be taken freely but potatoes and all farinaceous foods were to be strictly avoided. Vinegar was recommended to be taken only in moderation. To produce a lasting and gradual reduction in size the Cincinnati *Enquirer* declared that diet was of the greatest importance and with that and mild aperients an "unhealthy increase of adipose tissue may be prevented." With respect to exercise, said the piece, "To the stout woman exercise is generally a burden, but begun in small doses and increased gradually it will soon grow to be a pleasure and a benefit as well, if she is really determined to reduce her size."[23]

A reporter writing in the *Los Angeles Times* in 1896 declared that quick lunches made fat men after remarking that every person who acquired the quick-lunch habit got fat as soon as he had come under the regular influence of the system. Noting that men who had begun to acquire noticeable stomachs, and others with a disposition to stoutness, took on flesh rapidly, he said it was perfectly plain to see why it happened. Those daily luncheons, he argued, supplied bread, bread, and more bread, the most fattening thing a man could eat, unless it was the cakes and pastries that supplanted the bread. It was cheaper, he thought, for a man to get fat than to keep thin because if he confined himself "to such things as meat and salads, his luncheon costs him three or four times as much as it would if he would eat the sandwiches and the cakes..." Something had to be done to keep us from getting fat, he fretted, "because we cannot afford to pay for anything but doughnuts, sandwiches, cakes and milk."[24]

An 1896 story that originated in Wayne County, south of Canton,

Ohio, had it that the common poke or pokeberry that grew in the pastures or by the roadside in much profusion was a "certain cure" for obesity. It was said that if a "fat man will eat of them regularly, say a couple of quarts a day, he can reduce his flesh at the rate of ten pounds a week without feeling any discomfort and without altering his diet except to abstain from potatoes, bread and other fattening foods." That discovery was made by an area farmer who noticed that the birds that lived on the pokeberry patches were always very lean. He fed the berries to one of his hogs, as an experiment, and in a couple of weeks the animal was a skeleton. They had the same effect on chickens and finally, being obese himself, the farmer began to eat them. Within a month after starting to eat pokeberries he had reduced his weight more than 25 pounds and after that outcome some of his neighbors adopted the same cure with similar results.[25]

According to the New York *Tribune* in 1896, a great many women, convinced "that flesh is inimical to beauty — is the death blow to grace — injure health in the endeavor to reduce weight." And, "They put themselves to great trouble and inconvenience, swallow all sorts of preventives and remedies in order to get thin and then stand aghast at the spectacle of their wrinkled, flabby faces and throats, the result of the falling away of flesh under the elastic skin." For those willing to diet, the piece recommended they regulate their day as follows: a tumbler full of hot water must be taken on waking in the morning; "rise early and have a tepid bath, with vigorous brushing afterward with a flesh brush; and have only three meals a day with an avoidance of drinking at meals. Breakfast was to be one small cup of tea, some dry toast, boiled fish or a small cutlet, and a baked apple or a little fresh fruit. For the noon meal, white fish or meat, dry toast or stale bread, vegetables and fruit, either fresh or stewed. And for supper the meal recommended was toast, salad, fruit and six ounces of wine or water, "Hot water with lemon juice in it is good for supper."[26]

Two years later, in 1898, an article raised the possibility that within the next year or so we would have seaweed on our tables as a regular article of diet — that it was to be the next big fad — used as a relish as were lettuce and radishes. However, it was admitted that seaweed would never become a staple article of food in American diets "owing to its indigestibility." Touted as the variety of seaweed most likely to take hold was the focus vesiculosus, which was said to be an efficient remedy for obesity. One authority on algae reportedly said that if that were the variety used as the basis for an anti-fat remedy it would mean thousands of dollars to the manufacturer "and a proportionate falling off in flesh among those affiliated with a superabundance of fatty tissue."[27]

Mrs. S. T. Rorer wrote in the July 1898 issue of *Ladies' Home Journal* about the best foods for stout women. Best meats for the obese, she wrote, were beef, mutton, venison, and game, while the best fish were sole, flounder, cod, halibut, and white fish. Not desirable were the mollusk and the crustacean. Among vegetables the best were cauliflower, broccoli, the ordinary cabbage, kale and spinach, lettuce, endive, chicory, celery, turnips without sauce, artichokes, squash, cooked cucumbers, cress, very young green peas, and string beans. Best fruits were grapes, ripe peaches, raspberries, blackberries, strained and made into mush, and an occasional baked apple. Almonds and pine nuts were the best choices from the nut family. Other advice from Rorer included, "Dry toast made from whole wheat bread may form the basis of many delightful sandwiches for the noonday meal. Where the habit is to have a midday dinner, and supper in the evening, these sandwiches with a glass of half milk and half barley water, may form the supper. A glass of cool water may be taken on retiring." Rorer said the first meal of the day should be taken at noon sharp and consist of: two well-broiled chops or sweetbreads, or eggs in any form; one slice of well-baked whole wheat bread, buttered and thoroughly masticated; and one green vegetable; for dessert a cup of custard, or fruit — grapes, peaches, oranges, or baked apples. For the evening meal Rorer advised having a clear soup, a red meat (in fact, any meat except pork and veal), a succulent vegetable like spinach or cooked celery, a little lettuce, new peas, string beans, a little raw cabbage, or well-cooked cauliflower. All meat consumed was to be broiled, roasted or boiled — not fired. A half-pound of meat could be taken at the evening meal and dessert could consist of a piece of well-toasted whole wheat bread without butter, a bit of well-ripened cheese, and a cup of clear coffee. "The success of this treatment lies in doing without breakfast," Rorer explained. "The patient may eat sufficient to satisfy hunger but no more; in a few days she will find that the so-called hunger is not felt at the pit of the stomach, and in less than a week she will enjoy the two meals a day — the first at noon and the last at 5 or 6 o'clock — better than she has enjoyed her three meals."[28]

According to an unnamed New York physician commenting in 1898, with the coming of the warm weather every summer he got a flock of visits from women who wanted to get thin. "I may jog along in comparative peace all the winter and spring, working and praying with hysteria and prostration and neurasthenia and anemia and other simple and soulful complaints, but just as soon as the warm days come and I begin to promise myself a little rest and relaxation, in pops Mrs. A. with an anxious face and fifty or sixty pounds for which she has no use and sets about bargaining with me as if I were a Shylock," he explained. When such a patient came in asking him to reduce her obesity, he added, "I tell her to row a boat and take a ten-mile walk at 5 o'clock every morning. I warn her against catnaps, cool drinks, green peas and all the other pleasures of life, and she goes away radiant. She always loses five or ten pounds during the summer, often more."[29]

Also in 1898, an article in *Scientific American* declared that obesity could be successfully cured by a fruit diet and "this is due to the fact that fruit is a natural food and thus aids the system to establish a normal tissue metamorphosis and a normal balance between the processes of assimilation and dissimilation, but also because it affords a very comfortable means of reducing the amount of nutrient material received to a minimum quantity." According to the piece, the writer had succeeded in reducing excessive weight "in the most satisfactory manner by prescribing a diet consisting almost exclusively of grapes or apples, allowing only a small bit of thoroughly dried bread or zwieback in connection with the fruit."[30]

An article that first appeared in *Harper's Bazaar* in 1899 proclaimed that while general exercise was valuable in fighting obesity "it is not sufficient to aid those who are too stout, particularly those annoyed by embonpoint, but specific notions are necessary." He suggested a simple exercise that worked "wonders." The person was to stand erect with her heels together and arms at her side (corsets and long skirts had to be absent). Then the person was to touch the floor in front of the feet with the fingertips, without bending the knees, and then to repeat the procedure 15 times. "This simple exercise has been known to reduce the weight twenty pounds in three months, the greatest effect being over the abdomen," went the account. When it came to recommendations of a diet for obesity, said the article, "the rules are so much like those for dyspepsia and gout that invalidism is suggested. Primarily the ban goes out against that wicked trio of sweets, fats and starches. All are tabooed and that means a diet so monotonously simple that many a one lapses into her former state of indulgence from weariness and impatience." In that diet there could be no candy, "no enticing drinks from the soda-water fountain," no sugar in tea and coffee (saccharine was allowed), no desserts, nor could there be anything fried, no mayonnaise, no creamy things, no farinaceous items, vegetables that grew below the ground such as potatoes and beets had to be omitted from this diet, and butter was forbidden. What was left was the following: "A cup of hot water an hour before meals, none with food; fresh meats — except pork — and pulled bread, with some indulgence in vegetables and fruit. This, of course, is severe, but it is only necessary for a short time and will surely lower the weight. After a sufficient number of pounds have vanished into thin air, a more generous diet should be gradually adopted."[31]

Giving advice to fat people in 1902, an unnamed Washington, D. C., physician declared that spring was the best time for fat people to try to reduce their weight. That was so because in the first place, a person could get better substitutes for articles of food that were regarded as "flesh producers," and a person could take exercise with a greater degree of enjoyment. Then he outlined a "heroic" treatment for obesity the French tried in the spring and one he considered to be one of the least harmful of such methods. It consisted of eating spinach in large quantities and a moderate amount of rare broiled beefsteak. The French called spinach the "broom of the stomach" and the medical man called it undoubtedly a "great vegetable for dyspeptics." This doctor argued that a good number of fat people looked healthy but in reality suffered from dyspepsia. With respect to the diet of spinach and beefsteak the physician said, "It allows little latitude to the patient, who must partake of the diet three times a day, with the possible exception of breakfast, when toast and coffee may be substituted." Under this regimen, he reminded his readers, nothing that contained sugar was to be eaten, although saccharine was allowed to those who desired something sweet. Water was not to be taken with meals but as much water as possible should be drunk between mealtimes, provided at least an hour had elapsed since eating. Add to that diet plenty of exercise and the obesity cure will be "rapid and not unpleasant." Spinach, he added, also had a "wonderful effect in clearing up the complexion."[32]

In the annals of individuals who had effected dramatic weight losses was the well-known Washington, D. C., druggist Dr. E. M. McComas who in 1902, when he was 50, had lost 207 pounds but, nevertheless, was still described as being "far from trim." Six years earlier he weighed 417 pounds but was down to 210 pounds in January 1902. He explained, "Six years ago my life was a burden. I was almost useless to myself and to everyone else. I was a sight — a monstrosity — a human elephant. People came to my store just to see me. I had been fat since childhood." McComas said, "Fat people because of their size are apt to become indifferent to things and live an indolent life. I had fallen into this way. I sat on a chair nearly all day. It was too uncomfortable and was too much trouble to move around, and as for walking, I never walked." Even a distance of two blocks was too much for him to walk and if he had to go that distance he took a streetcar. He had not been downtown for years and when he got into a streetcar he took up the room that three people generally occupied. "When I walked up a flight of stairs, which was done with the greatest of effort, it took me ten minutes to regain my breath. I had not taken a good, long breath in years." As his breath got shorter and shorter he came to the conclusion that he would some day drop dead from fatty degeneration of the heart. He had gotten so obese that he could not sleep lying down but had to sleep in a chair. It was at that point that he determined to get thin enough so he could lie down at night to sleep like other people.[33]

McComas studied the literature on obesity and concocted several mixtures of medicine, the last of which supposedly worked. He took that medication (no details of the preparation were revealed) for a year, combined with changes to his diet, and then stopped taking the preparation, relying on diet alone. During the first six months of his reducing regime, he said, he ate only four meals during the first month, one meal per week. After one month he had lost 50 pounds; then he took up walking and commenced to eat one meal a day. "I never have been much of a vegetable eater, but live mostly on bread and butter and meats. I was careful not to eat pastry and farinaceous foods, but other than this did not follow any particular diet," he said. Concluded McComas, "Many persons have expressed surprise that the loss of my fat did not leave me wrinkled, but it did not, and this does away with a pet theory advanced by so many ladies who hesitate to attempt any anti-fat for fear of wrinkles."[34]

Ella Fletcher discussed the effort to appear slender in a lengthy 1902 news account, noting firstly, "The taking on of flesh until it becomes a burden is a self-inflicted evil, oftener than otherwise generated by enervating ease and luxury. So insidious are the advances of this cormorant obesity that its victims seldom take alarm promptly." She regarded obesity as a disease of "malassimilation" and, "Overindulgence in sweets, pastries and cakes, rich entrees and all the tempting starchy foods which are given such prominence on our extravagant American tables is usually the originating cause of obesity." Fletcher felt it was natural that the stout person was disinclined to activity, "for no shackles are more burdensome than superfluous pounds of flesh that make every step a weariness, every movement, even, an effort, and crowd upon your lungs and heart, impeding breath and circulation to the point of acute discomfort. These shackles weigh also as heavily upon the mind and will power as upon the physique and render the body a tyrant." A wise woman would never shut herself up in such a prison of flesh, Fletcher warned, for she not only deprived herself of the joys of an active life, but also sacrificed her beauty to the encroaching flesh and jeopardized her health and happiness. "She should take alarm the moment any part of her body gains unduly, for every additional pound of flesh beyond that which rounds out the form to harmonious proportions is a menace to her beauty, health and usefulness," she added.[35]

With respect to clothing, Ella Fletcher argued it was a mistake to attempt to restrain the encroaching flesh by tying the corset strings tighter, for that only made a bad situation worse. But she described the straight front corset, when properly worn without exaggeration, as a boon to the victim of obesity. It was said to have been an expedient devised by Mlle. Calve, when she returned to America after a two-year absence, with an increase of flesh that almost "burst the bounds of decorum." Calve started a fashion that was soon copied the world over. When there was an oversupply of fatty atoms in the blood, explained Fletcher, nature was perplexed to find storage for them, and wherever the circulation was weakish or rendered sluggish by compression nature deposited them abundantly. Warning signs were described by Fletcher as follows; "The first indication of the abdomen taking upon itself undue prominence usually is accompanied by the discomfort of a sensation of fullness after eating and shortness of breath, and this is the moment when a woman still can refuse to become a prisoner to corporeal conditions. Slight changes of diet and mode of life at this time would correct its progress and save suffering."[36]

Fletcher said the first step to the cure of obesity was to implement changes in the habits of life, which caused it, with exercise an important part of the regime. Sedentary occupations and driving had to give way to active outdoor exercise when possible and a system of physical movement had to be practiced morning and night. It was important that the corpulent woman learned to sit and stand correctly and that she "acquaint herself with the relaxed muscles and nerves of the abdomen, so that she can restrain them to their normal duty." Then she advised five minutes of exercise each morning and night while lying on one's back, contrasting and expanding those abdominal muscles. "Deep breathing is of importance for obesity sufferers, as it increases combustion, which demands fat for fuel; therefore breathing exercises should precede all others and should alternate with them." Also, Fletcher recommended working out with Indian clubs. As regarded diet, Fletcher felt an "immoderate" appetite had to be restrained but the kind of food eaten was more important than the quantity. Midnight suppers of rich food and between-meal snacks, together with all dainties and sweets, had to be relinquished. Bread was to be eaten sparingly and only of the coarse kinds — gluten, graham, and whole wheat. No white bread was to be taken, except in the form of thin, crisp toast. Potatoes, beans, peas and corn were the "mischief-breeding" vegetables and had to be shunned completely, along with all forms of Italian pastes. However, wholesome greens and salads were the "fleshy woman's friend," and offered sufficient variety to pique the appetite. All kinds of meat except pork and veal could be eaten and most fish; but salmon, sardines, mackerel and eels were on the blacklist as fat-producing items. Of soups, only small portions of clear consommé were allowed. "It is an idiosyncrasy of obesity that its victims are afflicted with a consuming thirst, and restraint in the matter of drink is the greatest trial of their reduction regime," said Fletcher. "The chief evil is from drinking freely during the meal and this habit must be broken gradually." For a week or two a glass of white wine diluted with Vichy was permitted but later, except for weak tea or coffee for breakfast, all drink had to be taken before and after meals, and hot water was preferable to cold. Chocolate, old or sweet wines and all malt beverages were "fat-producing" and thus placed on the blacklist by Fletcher, as were bananas, grapes, peaches, prunes, and melons. However, most other fruits could be eaten abundantly.[37]

Physician Dr. W. Latson argued in 1903 that measures to treat obesity could be divided into two classes: a) general or constitutional, and b) local. For example, in the first class, the amount of food consumed should be reduced to a quantity commensurate with the assimilative capacity of the individual, "This will often necessitate also an increase in the amount of physical exercise taken. In other words the man or woman who would reduce to symmetrical proportions an obese body must first establish a physiologic balance between the food taken and the work done. In many mild cases no treatment further than this will be necessary. Halve the food; double the work." In many other cases, though, more work was necessary, he argued, as perhaps there was a habit of taking an excess of fluids with meals. "The safest rule on this matter is perhaps the following: Take not more than one pint of fluids with a meal and never take fluid into the mouth while it contains food." Latson stated the eating of pastry and candy was a common cause of obesity and while he praised wheat and fruit as wholesome, nutritious foods, he deplored the way they were put to use to make fruit pies. "When these ingredients, however, are subjected to the processes necessary to make a pie or a pudding they are not only quite impoverished from a dietetic standpoint but are an actual injury to the system, affecting it in many ways," explained Latson. "One of these is to produce obesity."[38]

Diet was important to reduce obesity, declared Latson, and he argued that many mistakes had been made in the past. The old plan of eliminating from the diet the carbohydrates — that is, the starches and sugars — he described as "absurd and pernicious." As a general rule he advised two meals a day with the first meal to consist of fruit alone, or fruit with whole wheat bread, or fruit with cereal and milk. As to the second meal, it could be made up of three or four simple articles of food such as peas, beans, baked potatoes, salad, fruit, and cereal, "Meat, if desired, can be taken in place of the beans or peas, but is rather less desirable for several reasons." Among food items to be avoided were spices, condiments, and sauces with tea, coffee, and tobacco to be used sparingly, if at all. Alcohol was best avoided altogether. "While an excess of fluids with meals is to be avoided, yet the free use of water between meals and on rising and retiring is helpful in obesity, since it increased elimination," added Latson. "The amount of water taken daily should not be less than two quarts." He stressed the need for exercise and thought that very often vigorous exercise alone without any other measure was sufficient to reduce the obese body to symmetry. Running, swimming, boxing, riding, golf, tennis, and boating were all recommended as good exercises. For local treatment of obesity Latson recommended specific exercises for fat deposits on specific parts of the body.[39]

Articles advising people to deal with obesity through exercise alone were few and far between in this period; most dealt with diet alone while a few added a relatively few words of advice on exercise to their main focus of diet. One of the exceptions was a piece that appeared in *McCall's Magazine* early in 1903. According to the introduction, the subject of the cure of obesity "is one which has personal interest for a very large number of people, especially those middle-aged persons who have a tendency to the increase of adipose deposit. Diet systems of cure almost always fail because patients seldom have the patience to persevere long enough with a dietetic regime, or because they do not carry it out in its entirety." Diet regimes could also be difficult to follow when one was away from home, as normal eating conditions were not available, and so on. But those drawbacks did not apply to physical exercises, argued the piece, although it admitted the disadvantage of many physical exercises was that they made too great a demand upon the strength and energy. Reportedly, a famous (but unnamed) medical doctor had made a special study of physical culture and continued movements of the muscles (that led to a muscular development not socially acceptable then in women) was not necessary to achieve the result of curbing obesity. Rather, vibration of the muscles did all the work required, "without the evil results so often following over-exercise." Thus, this article advised a system that consisted in tensing the muscles as hard as possible, "and then to vibrate them strenuously for a minute. Nothing more is required, and a few minutes of such work every day is guaranteed to give greater chest expansion, development, and solidity of muscle than any other system, while at the same time burning away, as it were, superfluous flesh — that is to say, getting rid of the unhealthy, flabby tissue, and reducing the obese person to graceful and healthy proportions." Paradoxically, said the article, the exercises were equally useful for increasing flesh on thin people. By making use of six separate movements it was said to be possible to exercise every muscle of the trunk and limbs. Then the article gave the six exercises in detail, most were gentle stretching exercises. For example, number three went as follows, "With the arms stretched out on either side, bend the body at the hips very slowly until one hand points directly upward and the other downward. Remain in this position for a few seconds, breathing deeply, then go to the other extreme." In conclusion, went the piece, "The exercises [all six] should not be prolonged for more than five minutes. Four or five minutes given to them twice a day, morning and evening, is sufficient."[40]

A month or so later another article appeared on exercise alone, in the newspaper. Readers were advised not to neglect exercise but not to overdo it because "Too much exercise will alone set up obesity, because it weakens the whole digestive apparatus. Doctors don't seem to think of this, but it is so. Many a bicycle 'scorcher' has actually increased his adipose tissue." Among the best exercises for women were skipping, badminton, and lawn tennis, "The first is excellent for the tendency to abdominal obesity to which they are so liable; the second and third are good generally, because they put in action all parts of the body." Walking and scrubbing (housework) were also noted as being good for keeping down fat. For men the best exercises were given as baseball, cricket, football and golf. And for both sexes, generally, "Light dumbbell or Indian club exercise will do good, and nothing is better as a fat-preventer than a short, brisk walk before breakfast."[41]

Journalist Katherine Morton produced a long article on the topic in 1906, targeted at women as newspapers and magazines increasingly directed stories on obesity to women only, over and above those aimed at the entire general population. Morton declared that English writers told that the American idea of beauty involved females weighing more than that acceptable by the strict canons of beauty, "but the English writer knows nothing of the struggle of our women against the ever increasing layers of adipose tissue induced by the luxuries and conveniences of up-to-date modern life. American women of the leisure class certainly tend to increase in weight, as they grow older. They walk less than other women in the world, as a rule, and the veranda habitué is only seen in our country and in the tropics. In both places the woman rapidly acquires the too solid flesh and then wishes she hadn't." She acknowledged that reducing one's weight required much perseverance and self-denial since it necessitated abstinence from many "of the petty indulgences which have induced the unpleasant condition. Fat itself is an accumulation of unburnt and unconsumed body fuel: in other words, fat is carbon, and carbon is consumed by oxygen, which we inhale through our lungs." The reason that rapid walking, bicycle riding, and so on, reduced the flesh, explained Morton "is that during the practice of these the blood is rapidly oxygenized, and the result is the destruction or the burning out of the fat. People who live in high altitudes, or who are great walkers, are never fat." In her view the greatest flesh producers were sleep, lack of physical activity, sugar and starchy foods, and the stout woman usually had a decided disinclination to sacrifice on any of those points.[42]

The first step the stout woman should take, advised Morton, was to limit herself to a maximum of seven hours sleep, and no mid-day naps. When she arose in the morning a cold sponge bath was advised and the wealthy woman was to indulge in an "anatomical scrub"— that was a combination bath and rub administered by a "scientific" Swedish masseuse. The masseuse scrubbed off the flesh as she rubbed the muscles and manipulated the tissues with her brushes and "Particular attention is given to massaging — or I should say, scrubbing away — the double chin, the first sign of overripe maturity." According to Morton, a tight collar was the cause of more double chins than anything else. After the daily bath the woman who wished to regain her once slender figure should devote "a few moments" to exercises. It was noted that actor Lillian Russell, whose fight with the enemy of beauty — flesh — had become almost a national interest, could bend at the waist, touching the floor with her fingers without bending the knees, even in her street clothes. Women who objected to "violent exercises" were told to use a pomade that would reduce the size of her hips. That pomade was made as follows, and was applied to the fatty parts of the body: three grams iodine of potassium; 50 grams of vasoline; 20 drops, tincture of benzoin; 50 grams of lanoline; and while using that remedy the person was told to abstain from all fat-forming foods as far as possible. Women who wished to lose weight rapidly were told to wrap themselves in rubber bandages — which were made especially for this purpose — and, wearing those heavy garments, take violent exercises until they were in a dripping perspiration, "for the flesh literally melts off, but it is not to be recommended where the patient is at all delicate or suffering from any form of heart trouble. However, the rubber suits are being made for some of our best known women, and they certainly work a lightning change in one's appearance."[43]

With respect to diet, Morton advised the stout woman to eliminate from her menu all hot wheat breads, potatoes, pastry of every sort and sugar. Saccharine tablets were allowed to be used to sweeten coffee. Oil and butter were also denied to the dieter; toast was substituted for the morning roll. All ripe fruit, except bananas, were recommended but meat had to be limited to under-done steaks or mutton. Eggs were allowed, as were vegetables such as cabbages, tomatoes, cucumbers, turnips, and beets. And, "Deep breathing exercises and long walks and bicycle rides must be taken, at least two miles first and later, more, every day by the woman who wishes to reduce — no matter whether she puts her trust in the efficacy of the rubber suit or the mechanical massage. All of these are excellent accessories but they are merely aids, and should not be depended on entirely for the reduction of flesh."[44]

According to a story in the *Washington Post* in 1907 it was said there were too many fat people and too many thin people in the United States and the federal government, through the Agriculture Department, was conducting experiments to bring both groups back to normalcy. Nutritional investigations were then underway as well as experiments being conducted by the government in how to make people thin, or fat. All of those federal government efforts were taking place at the University of Maine at Orono and at the University of Tennessee at Knoxville. Said a government spokesman, "Now is the time to get thin. With the approach of the summer and its green vegetables the path of the fat man who wants to reduce is made easy." To the fat man who wanted to get thin, the government said, "Eat little, sleep little, and drink less." To the thin man who wanted to gain weight the government declared, "Drink all you can, eat all you can, and sleep as much as you can." An Agriculture Department spokesman pointed out that summer was the season of the year when people who were "inconvenienced" by fat could easily get rid of some of it. The heat of the summer naturally tended to reduce the weight, for it caused perspiration, and that meant the discharge of a good deal of water under the skin. But the principal inducement of summer was that the season offered many fresh vegetables such as tomatoes, onions, lettuce, radishes, and so on, "which the fat man may eat by the wholesale with impunity."[45]

According to the story the course prescribed for the fat man who wanted to become thin was especially trying because it meant giving up the "good things in life." He was not to drink a drop of water or any other kind of liquid one hour before eating or before one hour had elapsed after he had finished eating. And if he could go without liquid for two hours before and for two hours after eating it was even more beneficial. Breakfast had to consist of eggs, toast, and coffee or cocoa, without sugar while lunch was to be confined to a simple piece of meat or a cup of consommé or some fruit. For his supper the fat man reducing could have any kind of meat, in any quantity, and no vegetables other than tomatoes, spinach or cucumbers; no bread or butter was allowed. And while he was allowed a cup of tea it must contain no sugar. Also on the list of banned food items were peas, beans, beets, potatoes, cauliflowers, cabbages, parsnips, bananas, veal, and anything containing starch or sugar. He was expected to live mainly upon apples, oranges, grapes, other acid fruits and the three or four vegetables that tended to "thin the blood." Also, he was expected to drink no alcohol, no milk, and very little water. One glass of sour claret was allowed at supper, but no more. Agriculture Department experts said that after a month of such a course of action "a fat man will be able to look at himself with pride."[46]

A few weeks later another article summarized the federal government activity and its diet recommendations, and then went on to add a few tips of its own. Reportedly, there was nothing so effective in reducing weight as worry, but worry was a dangerous remedy as ill health was a boon companion to worry, so the article advised its readers to laugh and remain fat, rather than employ worry as a reducing agent. However, for the person in good health, they could "take on flesh by drinking much water. Hot water is productive of good results. There are half a dozen persons in Ogden [Utah] who have increased their weight twenty pounds each by drinking hot water and the increased flesh and the use of hot water have but added to their vigor."[47]

Typical of articles — with a tendency to increase in length — aimed at women only was a 1907 piece in the *Washington Post* titled, "Fifty ways for fat women to become thin." It chronicled the growing fad and trend of women turning to weight reduction. One of the "most celebrated of fat eradicators" (unnamed) declared that excessive plumpness was no longer fashionable adding that it was unnecessary and decidedly out of date. Years earlier, said the authority, when people got fat they looked on it as a dispensation of Providence, as they did on gray hair or baldness; in fact, they considered it a sort of hallmark of success. They had no way of getting rid of it so they did the next best thing and made the best of it. A happily married woman had three good, substantial meals with pie on the side every day and soon began to put on weight. Once started it was next to impossible to stop gaining weight. Those days from the past were described by the authority as "the days of rocking chairs — rocking chairs and fat. Now you can find women sixty years of age as slim as in their youth, without a rocking chair in the family, and with pie tabooed. Of course there is no doubt that we don't have as good a time as we used to have with plenty to eat and no one to look askance, but then we're thinner, and you can't have everything in this world. At the present time there are fifty ways of getting thin and only one of staying so. The one is briefly told in the word self-sacrifice."[48]

A second authority consulted on the subject by the *Post* reporter was a physician (also unnamed) of the Murray Hill neighborhood in New York City. He stated the secret of beauty was to find the weight a woman's height and bone size demanded and to then maintain it — below was anemia and above was shapelessness. "But to say that all women were intended to be thin is nonsense. Juno has her place in the world. But the trouble is that women will not find that special weight," said the physician. He thought that dressmakers furthered the "flesh-losing habit" by designing all their fashions for slim women, who for years had been depicting lean females. If fat were to come back into fashion tomorrow, he speculated, just about half a million people would have to go out of business; that is, there would be a financial panic for the beauty doctors, obesity curers, and so on, who made up a large portion of the community. From his point of view, he said with exaggeration, people could be divided into two classes — those who were taking flesh off and those who were having it taken off. Summer was a time that women dreaded, said the Murray Hill physician, because hot weather meant inaction, "and it may be stated that the average woman who is at all inclined to flesh puts on anywhere from five to ten pounds every season." If he were asked to give a simple recipe for taking off flesh, one that would not necessitate starving, an abnormal amount of exercise, or drugs, he would reply, "get a husband to worry over." The real problem arose, he stated, when a woman had to diet and was told to give up sweets, and "the matter of dieting is merely a matter of leaving out of your menu everything that you like. Sweets, rich dishes, gravies of all kinds are strictly tabooed. Then nothing must be drunk with the meals, especially alcohol in any form. It is necessary, as the French say, to suffer in order to be beautiful."[49]

The *Post* reporter put the question of exercise as a value in reducing flesh to several "experts" and found all conceded that there was no surer way of reducing superfluous flesh than by regular exercise combined with diet. Also, all conceded that woman, being at best an impatient creature, "is not as a general thing satisfied with the meager results shown from day to day. Women get stout gradually, but they want to get thin in a hurry. Men often take exercise merely for the pleasure of it; women rarely do." One of the diet and exercise promoters remarked that one of his main problems was to prevent women from throwing their whole regime over after a few weeks, losing their time and money while turning instead to some get-slim-soon quack remedy. At one of the city's Turkish baths the manager observed that never before in the 30 years of its existence had it been so overrun by patrons. "We can't begin to take care of them," she confessed. "Some of our patients take three or four a week. Where there used to be one woman bothering about her complexion there are a hundred now worrying about their figures." She added that one of the problems was that as soon as they emerged from the Turkish bath they ordered a cocktail or highball, available at the baths, because they were tired. But, of course, declared the manger, they could not lose weight under those circumstances.[50]

Dr. T. J. Allen was a physician with a medical advice newspaper column, one of many such doctors, in 1910. That year he pointed out that a man 5'8" in height should weigh about 154 pounds and a woman of that height should weigh five pounds less. Twenty pounds above or below that so-called normal indicated an abnormal condition of sufficient magnitude to warrant special attention, said Allen. For corpulence he said the natural and safest remedy was fasting, with proper safeguards; drugs were always to be avoided as agents of weight reduction. After a fast reduced the weight to normal, the tendency was to remain much below the former abnormal weight, although it might be necessary to repeat the fast at intervals of several months "before the habit of accumulating superfluous flesh is overcome."[51]

Non-medical advice on the topic of obesity came from Lina Cavalieri in her regular column, wherein could often be found the exaggerated by-line, "By Mme. Lina Cavalieri, the most famous living beauty." An editorial lead-in for a Cavalieri column in July 1911 said, "All women are interested in cures for superfluous flesh, the plump ones because they want to rid themselves of twenty, thirty, or forty pounds, the thin ones so that they may remain thin." Cavalieri exclaimed that she hoped all her overweight female readers had used the summer to lose weight because summer was "nature's fat cure" and even in late July it was not too late to turn the last warm weeks to advantage. Summer, she said, was the best reducing season for three "excellent" reasons: 1) in summer the amount of food consumed was reduced because the appetite was less robust; 2) in summer more water was drunk and that quickened perspiration; 3) the heat caused far more perspiration in summer than in winter and perspiration invariably reduced weight. Cavalieri offered tips on what the woman could do to help summer, such as by taking long walks in that warm weather season and to take them before breakfast. "A long brisk walk before breakfast, especially if you wear at such time a heavy woolen sweater to aid perspiration, and then stand under a shower or turn on a spray of cold, or at least cool water, to wash off the excretions from the pores, is an excellent beginning of the day by the woman who would grow thin," she explained.[52]

When it came to meals, Cavalieri declared she knew several women who had been successful in reducing who had contented themselves with a breakfast of three or four glasses of hot water to stave off hunger. For those who did eat a morning meal she advised that it be light and that the European breakfast was more wholesome than the American one; rolls, toast, and coffee with some fruit in season was described as quite enough. After breakfast, even if it was only hot water, readers were advised not to lounge around but to move about, perhaps by playing a game of golf or tennis or croquet. Or take another walk, at least for those on vacation. If not, then the exercise generated by the woman's household duties or by her business duties would substitute for what she had suggested for the vacationer. "The mental exercise in the one [business] tends almost as much toward reduction of weight as the physical exercise in the other," she said. One was to eat as little as possible for lunch, even if one was very hungry. Fruit, stewed rather than raw, a green salad with much vinegar and little oil, dry toast and meat (rare beef) with all particles of fat cut away, or two boiled or poached eggs were described as a nourishing but not fattening meal. No butter was allowed. For dinner there was to be more meat, as described above, more toast, a thin soup, a green salad of one vegetable such as asparagus or spinach, and more stewed fruit. Readers were told to "Drink nothing at meals." For hunger pangs between meals, Cavalieri advised her readers to take two or three cups of weak tea, without cream or sugar, to ease those gnawing aches. Before retiring for the night it was permitted to drink two or three glasses of hot water.[53]

Cavalieri added that she was "opposed to the starving which is a form of torture to which some apply the term dieting. I do not believe the stomach should long remain empty." She believed the gastric juices had to have something to work on and if there was no food then those juices went to work on the lining of the stomach. As well, she thought a fast could be useful in weight reduction once in a while, with the extreme limit for a fast being 48 hours. With respect to bathing, Lina declared, "Intelligent bathing is an aid in reduction. If Turkish baths are accessible two a week or one every other day will help greatly in reduction." For ordinary, everyday bathing she advised her readers "to make the baths your aid. Tepid baths, while better, in my opinion for the general health than either hot or cold baths, are aids to the formation of fat. Make your baths cooler, if not quite cold. Such baths harden the muscles and, by making the flesh more solid, reduce the bulk even though the weight may not considerably change." Concluded Cavalieri, "The use of a gentle laxative is a part of the most thorough reduction systems. Take only so much sleep as your require for strength building, for its is true that we fatten while we sleep."[54]

A couple of months later Lina returned with another lengthy column on the subject. In this one she offered reducing tips after expounding her bizarre theory that the causes of superfluous flesh in the woman of 30 and the woman of 40 were different. According to Lina when a woman between 25 and 30 began to acquire plumpness she supposed that those additional and pronounced curves were a sign of health and that impression was reinforced by insincere persons who said to her face, "How well you are looking" and then said to her back, "Isn't she getting a sight?" Even her doctor was said to not want to risk his fees by offending her with reference to her increasing fatness and the warning that what she regarded as signs of health were really symptoms of disease. For women like that, those in the 20 to 30 year-old range the cause of rapidly taking on flesh, said Cavalieri, was one of the following: 1) "suralimentation," which was merely indigestion; 2) latent dyspepsia; or 3) pre-existing nervousness. The cure for such women was a proper diet, consisting chiefly of vegetables and fruits, and frequent baths in cold or cool water. If the woman was a nervous person she was advised to eat her meals regularly, letting nothing interfere with them. But to eat very slowly, reducing the food to a liquid state in the mouth. "Stop the over-eating, which is a bad habit of the nervous person addicted to plumpness. Teach yourself that it is not masculine to be muscular. Train yourself to enjoy exercise. Exercise for a few days or weeks at a regular time, and the exercise will come to be a necessity. Exercise will make you healthier, as well as thinner, especially if you are of gouty or rheumatic tendency...And exercise out of doors is of twice the value of exercise indoors, for it permits oxygen to do its work of burning up the fat. Golf and tennis; rowing and long walks, are the best friends of the woman who would reduce 'thirty fat.'"[55]

For the woman aged 40 or so, argued Cavalieri, the cause of excess flesh was usually due to nervous troubles. Strange as it might seem to the casual observer, she said, the fat person was usually very nervous, especially when it was a middle-aged woman. As a result of that nervousness she had some form of indigestion; gastric, intestinal, or relating to the liver. Recommended as a cure for this group was "the practice of muscle cure...exercises with pulleys" limited to four pounds and "For the solid 'forty fat' bending at the waist is absolutely necessary. This flesh is more solid than that of the younger woman, and to banish it requires more persistence." After giving specifics for a few bending exercises she added, "Always bathe after these exercises. As I have always said, a bath should always follow perspiration. If you cannot endure a cold shower or spray or plunge, get into a tub of tepid water and let the water gradually run colder." A woman driving away "forty fat" could not endure the hard dietary restrictions imposed on the younger woman, said Lina, but she should eat temperately and no more than she was sure she actually needed. For the younger woman, dieting was to be the element most relied upon while for the older woman that element was to be muscle treatment, or exercise. Massage was recommended as an aid for both. General conclusions and recommendations by Cavalieri for both groups of women were for them to eat crackers instead of bread and eat no soup and drink neither beer nor wine. Household work was good for both groups and "So is stair and ladder climbing, and all exercises which cause you to step. When you are in the country, never lose an opportunity to climb a fence."[56]

Acting superstar Lillian Russell delivered advice to women on the topic of keeping fat at bay, in a 1913 newspaper article. She considered age to be an important factor with people seldom becoming fat before reaching the age of 40 and that women were more likely to become fat than were men. Thus, to avoid obesity it was necessary to take precautions as early middle life approached and that those precautions were especially necessary for women. One preventive measure consisted of limitation on food intake from the age of 30 to 35 years onward. Sugar and starchy foods (such as potatoes, bread, and rice) were to be eaten moderately, as were butter and other fats. Alcohol, especially beer, was to be avoided. Salt was to be used sparingly and liquids were to be taken between meals, never at them. Exercise was recommended and, said Russell, "There is no reason why any healthy woman shall not play tennis and golf, cycle and take part in other sports well into late middle life" and "Cold baths are of great service, but after the age of 35 they must be taken only with the approval of the physician. Turkish baths are also helpful, but here again, it is well to have medical advice." Suppose a person arriving at the "threatening" age was already fat? What was to be done? "It should be remembered that a fat person is also a weak person, and in certain cases the heart may be weak. Judicious treatment is therefore required. Indeed what a fat person needs is stimulation of the energies. The first measure is to regulate the diet." Russell went on to declare, "I have a system that works like magic. I can reduce myself or fatten myself within three days as I like." To reduce herself, for breakfast she had fruit, some toast, and a cup of tea or coffee; for lunch it was one chop, some salad, and a cup of tea without sugar or milk. "I drink nothing which contains alcohol and drink all the water I wish between meals."[57]

Grand opera singer Mme. Ernestine Schumann-Heink stated, at the start of 1913, that in the previous six months she had reduced her weight over 30 pounds, from 216 down to 179 pounds. Meat was said to be the secret for she only ate it once a month "to prove she is not a vegetarian." She said, "We eat too much meat: I owe the reduction to lemon juice, grapefruit, hard work, worry and abstinence from meat."[58]

In the October 1913 issue of *Women's Home Companion*, William J. Cromie, instructor at the University of Pennsylvania, had an article titled "Keeping a Good Figure" in which he said, "Many overstout women indulge too frequently in starchy foods, condiments, oily and highly-seasoned foods, sugar and liquids. The corpulent woman should never indulge in intoxicating liquors on account of their fat-producing properties, and because they lower vital resistance to disease." He favored water as the "natural drink" and that it should be taken between meals.[59]

Also in 1913, Dr. Gallsch, an English physician (who subscribed to the idea that sleep fattened), came up with a new treatment for obesity. Under his new dietary plan breakfast was a cup of tea with buttered bread; at 10 A.M. one egg was consumed with a small piece of bread and butter; at 1 P.M. lunch consisted of meat, vegetables, salad, and compote. In the afternoon coffee was taken with a little biscuit or white bread and butter while in the evening, supper consisted only of a small piece of bread and butter. According to a reporter, "the whole idea of the treatment is that it is the food taken in the evening and followed by the repose of night which particularly contributes to the formation of adipose tissue. Dr. Gallsch's patients invariably lose one or two pounds a week."[60]

Running over three days as a series in December 1913, and featured prominently in the *Los Angeles Times* was a series of articles with non-medical advice — hints to fat ladies — given by a trainer said to be well-known in the professional boxing world, identified only as "Abdul the Turk." Supposedly that series was published in response to fat ladies being conned by bogus cures. According to the lead-in, "To be a fat lady is a cruel fate. To be bunked is a sad experience. But to be bunked because you are a fat lady is almost too much for words. So the [newspaper] is coming to the rescue of the fair but fat charmers who are now besieging the Federal grand jury clamoring for revenge against 'God's Masterpiece' who sold them something that alleged to make them thin without effort." It was said the people who knew best how to get somebody thin were prizefight trainers and that was because they always got a fighter to weigh an exact, specified amount at an exact and specified point in time. And of all the boxing trainers the most expert was said to be Abdul the Turk, a man who had trained most of the prominent fighters of the time. Abdul even told the reporter he would reveal all, down to the point of telling the secret ingredient in his rubbing lotion, "For the sake of the poor bunked fat ladies." Said Abdul, "there is no easy way to take off flesh. Any one who tells you so is trying to feed you bunk. Anything that takes off your flesh except through your pores by hard work will do you harm. You can get thin by starving, or you can get thin by taking pills. But it will wreck your health. However, I can outline a plan whereby any woman, moderately strong, can take off from three to five pounds a week." All she had to do was eat what Abdul told her and do the exercises exactly as he detailed them.[61]

Part two of the series saw Abdul give his first specific advice and instructions. He began, "Fat lady, arise at 6:30 o'clock this morning. There is no hope for the fat lady who lies abed. In training fighters we always make calculations for their gaining weight over night. Sleep is the greatest fattener in the world. At 7:30 o'clock — one hour after getting up — the fat lady should have breakfast." She had to eat exactly what he prescribed, and at the exact time he said. Breakfast was to be prunes; a baked apple or grapefruit; two boiled eggs; toast; and tea. After breakfast a two hour rest was prescribed, during which time she could write letters or do light housework. Then she was to go for a walk, wearing the following, "warm woolen underclothing, heavy skirt, sweater" and to walk briskly for 25 minutes. On returning home she was to remove all her clothes and wrap herself up completely in a heavy army blanket in order to induce perspiration. After lying in the blanket for a few minutes she was to take a cold bath (slightly heated if she could not stand a cold bath). Then came the rub. "This is one of the most important features of the routine. We sometimes rub off from a quarter to half a pound at one time from fighters," explained Abdul. If she could afford it "the fat lady should have the rubbing done by a maid or a professional masseuse. The rub should last ten or fifteen minutes." If she could not afford to hire a masseuse then the woman was advised to rub herself with a coarse Turkish towel. At that point he revealed the secret formula for his special rubbing lotion — equal parts of alcohol, witch hazel, and eucalyptus oil. After the rub was finished the woman was to take a rest, a real rest, "Lie as though you were dead or were in a faint...Don't think of anything...Don't even think about growing thin. Don't read and don't talk." After 30 minutes of real resting the woman was to get up, get dressed and occupy the time until noon in light reading or some other light occupation. Lunch was to be a small piece of steak or a lamb chop; vegetables (never potatoes, which were to be avoided); and tea. No soft breads were permitted, but toast was allowed no pastry of any sort. That meal had to be taken at exactly noon every day, "These meal hours must not be varied one minute from the time I set forth," reiterated Abdul.[62]

Abdul allowed 2.5 hours of unstructured time after lunch but "Then begins the real grind of the day." His exercises were to be done in a gym if possible, or at home in the backyard, or inside in a big, open room. The woman was to wear tights and a heavy sweater, spend one minute on pulley weights (then rest for one minute); work out with dumbbells for three minutes; punch the bag for three rounds (two minutes of punching followed by one minute of rest for each round); skip rope for three minutes. "After this workout the fat lady should be perspiring profusely. After peeling off her tights she should have another cold bath and another. Then another relaxing rest," said the trainer. Dinner was taken at exactly 5:30 and consisted of steak or lamb chop, no greasy meat or greasy soup; dry bread or toast; non-starchy vegetables; tea; for dessert a little ice cream was permitted but no pastry or sweets of any kind. After dinner she was allowed to read or play cards, or even take a little walk but "The fat lady must prepare to go to bed at 9:30," said Abdul. Just before retiring she was to do light exercises for 15 minutes, such as thrashing her arms across her chest, bending over to touch her toes without bending her knees, and so on; then to bed.[63]

In Washington, D. C., The Congressional Lemon Club, in 1914, was not quite what its name implied, but an organization for the excessive consumption of lemons to reduce obesity. It was made up of women from the Congressional Club, many of them living at Congress Hall. One woman on the diet was said to have dropped from 188 pounds to 167 in two weeks. Under the regime an adherent took the juice of one lemon (straight) before breakfast on the first day; the juice of two lemons on the second day (not necessarily at the same time); three lemons on the third day, and so on, until 12 lemons were consumed in one day. Then the dieter went backwards, dropping one lemon each day, down to 11, to 10, and so on, down to the juice of one lemon a day, which was then to remain the permanent dose. No "cheating" with sugar or water was allowed and grape juice with the "medicine" was "absolutely prohibited." Lemons then sold for 35 cents a dozen at fashionable shops, ranging down to 18 cents at the unfashionable produce stands.[64]

Al Treloar was an executive at the Los Angeles Athletic Club and in late 1914 he initiated something new there, training tables — one for fat men to reduce on, and one for thin guys to build up on. That is, there were special menus for each group. According to a reporter, "It is a fact worthy of note that in the club membership are to be found many men whose amplitude is such that about the only thing they can buy ready made is a pocket handkerchief." He added that spinach, cabbage, lettuce, "and other luscious green vegetables which afford much exercise for the superior and inferior maxillaries and little satisfaction to the stomach are to form a staple diet for the heavies." It was also observed, "In order to reduce the mental anguish of the fats, Mr. Treloar has designed a special set of dishes which makes the meagerness of the menu less apparent. The plates and side dishes are all very thick and look as though they hold much more than their actual cargo. So when the luncheon comes on the fats do not at once realize the sum total of their woes." College athletes had the benefit of training tables, where their diet could be scientifically controlled, for many years by then, but the Los Angeles Athletic Club endeavor was said to be the first time the system was extended to an athletic club and to mature businessmen.[65]

A 1915 news account declared that over the course of time there appeared several dietary experts who had attained lasting fame through their "successful" treatments. Chief among them were Oertel, Ebstein, Banting, Schweninger, Schleicher, Germain, See, Hirschfield, and Von Noorden. Oertel's treatment was described as rather more liberal than the others and was well suited for those cases in which dietary changes could be combined with exercise. For exercise, Oertel prescribed a systematic course of hill climbing, and he greatly restricted the amount of fluid intake, contending that reduced blood pressure and lessened venous stasis. "The result claimed is that nutritive changes are produced in the fatty tissues which cause the food to become disintegrated, carried away and burned up," said the account. Oertel's system called for four meals a day and allowed the following items; lean roast and boiled beef, and veal, mutton, game and eggs. Spinach and cabbage were highly valued among the vegetables but fats and starches were restricted as much as possible. Sugar was banned completely. "The fluid prescribed consists of a moderate cup (about six ounces) of coffee or tea or milk twice a day, with 12 ounces of wine with an equal quantity of water, which may be taken at dinner," noted the journalist. "The amount of fluid allowed should not all be taken with meals, but at intervals during the day to allay the thirst." Water should never be allowed in quantity, said Oertel, and what little was allowed was to be consumed at intervals during the day. Although Oertel allowed a little wine he did so "simply because most of the Europeans demand it." In conclusion, stated the article, "Modern tests have proved beyond doubt that the entire absence of any kind of alcoholic beverages aids greatly in the reduction of flesh. Alcoholism is believed to be the inviting cause of some of the worst forms of obesity, especially that of a hereditary character."[66]

An article in the *Washington Post* in 1915 declared that medical treatment was hardly ever required to relive obesity. People in good health could decrease their weight without the aid of a physician. If a person was no more than 20 pounds overweight then the answer was systematic daily exercise in the open air with walking being called the simplest of all exercises for reducing the weight. Recommended was a daily five-mile walk as the surest and safest remedy for obesity. With respect to diet, readers were advised to remove all sweets and starches from their diets, and to eat very sparingly of roots and vegetables grown underground. It was recommended the diet be confined chiefly to meat (beef or mutton), fish, lettuce, celery, tomatoes, spinach, cucumbers, onions, watercress, cabbage, stale or toasted bread, and acid fruits. Peanuts were called an "excellent" article of food for the corpulent. "It should be borne in mind that an increase in flesh and weight is normal and natural in many families as they approach middle life," concluded the piece. "If one has been fat from childhood to middle age, to try to reduce the weight materially would be only at the expense of injury to the health."[67]

Under the weight reduction program that Dr. W. E. Preble of the Boston Dispensary medical staff had arranged in 1916 he had ruled out bread, alcoholic beverages, and sugar in any form, for the obesity class at the Dispensary. Fats of all kind were also completely tabooed. Preble did allow his obesity class members to eat all the potatoes they wanted, and eggs, a moderate amount of milk, all green vegetables, and meat and fish. As well, he refrained from barring or limiting water intake, being of the opinion that few people drank enough water. Although the reporter doing the story declared Preble's program for reducing weight had been "exceptionally successful" with some 40 women who had followed it for six months he later stated, "No actual record has been kept of the results, so that no actual figures can be procured." He also advised women in his program to take plenty of exercise, with the understanding being that women had plenty of opportunity to exercise while doing their housework and caring for children. Plenty of walking in the open air, good ventilation of their rooms at night and deep breathing were other requirements." Preble believed the chief causes of obesity "are the eating of sweets, rich food, too little exercise and occasionally the use of alcoholic drinks."[68]

Late in the summer of 1916, columnist Lina Cavalieri returned with another piece on the topic of obesity. Mostly it was a rehash of earlier advice. Summer was described as the best season of the year to lose weight and fat people were told to practice deep breathing because "The deep breathing person may be muscular, but is never fat." And, "Even the grossest stomach rejects much meat in the warm months of the year and longs for light grains and cooling vegetables and juicy fruits. These are the thinning foods and summer is the time to accustom oneself to them." The stout person, she said, shrank from the "muscle-hardening cold bath" but summer made it easy to take them.[69]

Physician Dr. Leonard Hirshberg was also the author of a health advice column. In 1919 he offered the opinion that a breakfast of coffee, toast, and fruit, without milk, sugar, or cream, was more than a fat person should have. He advised that alternate days without breakfast or nothing more than a cup of coffee made "hefty inroads upon your adipose fabric." After advocating brisk walks, Hirshberg declared, "A curious craving of the flesh of fat persons is for candies, cakes, sweets, dainties and the very articles, which, physically speaking, add insult to injury. Another set of habits conducive to obesity is riding in elevators, motor cars, street cars, subways and trains, when a brisk walk is exactly the antidote needed to reduce." He recommended his readers consume water in abundance, but not at mealtimes. "Massage and baths are also an undoubted aid in the reduction of flesh. This does not mean that massage should take the place of exercise but it should supplement exercise," he explained. "It has been estimated by experts that a thorough massage given by a skillful operator is equivalent to a seven-mile walk." Hirshberg did not recommend the cool or cold baths so many others did, at least not for women "as the delicate constitution of a woman is likely to be injured." Turkish baths were much better, he argued, but twice a week at most.[70]

Throughout this period dietary advice was always vague such as in the admonition to eat toast, consume some meat, and so on. That was because the precise measurement of caloric value of foods was barely underway, and that was a necessary step before dietary advice could be said to rest on scientific grounds. That is, a diet prescribing a certain number of calories per day for a person, and accurate knowledge of the caloric value of food items. Dr. Harry S. Greenbaum, instructor in medicine at Johns Hopkins University in Baltimore, surveyed the literature late in 1909 and found very little information listing caloric value of foods by the ounce, the best way to list them, he thought. His 1909 article did just that, listing food items in lengthy detail. As well, he gave the standards for American daily diets (from the U.S. Department of Agriculture). For example, a woman who performed light muscular work during her day needed 90 grams of protein (about three ounces) and 2,400 calories; a woman doing moderate muscular work needed 100 grams of protein and 2,700 calories; a man doing no muscular work needed 112 grams and 3,000 calories; a man doing moderate work required 125 grams and 3,500 calories; and a man doing hard muscular work needed 150 grams of protein daily, and 4,500 calories.[71]

Further evidence of a move to put the treatment of obesity, dieting, and remedies on a more scientific basis could be found in a 1915 article in *Literary Digest*, which declared, "One of the recent conquests of modern medicine is the application of remedial measures for obesity." That is, the treatment of obesity was moving beyond the purview of quacks only. Cited extensively in the article was Dr. William Brady, a medical superstar of the era. Brady said, "The time is approaching when no one will grow fat unless he is looking for an easy job with a side-show." He went on to say that people were stout mainly for two reasons, "The first is that they eat too much and exercise too little. The second, which is more important, is that there is some defect in their oxidation apparatus — some failure of certain of the ductless gland." One example he cited was deficient secretions in the pituitary gland. Brady added, "The most common type of obesity is merely a matter of excessive intake of fuel coupled with plain laziness. Let us hasten to add that laziness means, in this indictment, lack of real exercise." While much of what Brady said made sense and remains with us to this day as an appropriate analysis of the situation, much of what he said was nonsense. But it marked the transition that took place late in the 1880 to 1919 period as nonsense and quackery gave way to science and medicine. Among the nonsense delivered by Brady was that water should not be taken at mealtimes since cold water increased the secretion of gastric juices and that certain "types" of obesity were "certainly made much worse by much water-drinking." He favored eating vegetables that grew above the ground and the idea that eating just one kind of food at a meal was a good scheme.[72]

6

Style and Prevalence, 1880–1919

As early as 1880 reports of the prevalence of obese people began to surface. Mostly they were vague and anecdotal; there was no operational definition of obesity in use. According to a news account in March of that year, "It is said that America is becoming noted for the obesity of her women; therefore anti-fat remedies are sown broadcast over the land."[1]

Later that same year it was observed, "There are more fat women in Saratoga [New York, a fashionable resort area for the elite] than in any other place in this country at this time of year, and there is some talk of getting up a fat women's show." According to the report, several managers of dime museums had combined forces to travel to Saratoga to see if there was some plan they could implement to persuade "some of the fatties to put themselves on display." While they had talked quietly with the area hotel managers the latter doubted whether "their ponderous but beautiful guests will take part in any such show." Since most of those obese women were very wealthy offering them money to display themselves publicly had little incentive value. The reporter counted about 40 women lounging on the plaza of the Windsor Hotel and estimated 33 of them each weighed at least 200 pounds, while the Kensington Hotel was "noted" for its fat women and if there were any thin ones there they were in hiding. Thinnest of the women this reporter saw upon the plaza of the Kensington he estimated to have weighed 185 pounds. Congress Hall was said to have claimed to have more fat women than any other hotel in the two hemispheres. Of 91 women on the plaza of that hotel, the reporter estimated that only four of them could have weighed less than 190 pounds. At the Union Hotel he found 100 "of the loveliest and fattest ladies in the land." And, he remarked, "At the United States Hotel the proprietors have distributed all over the plazas and gardens weighing machines where the ladies may drop a nickel and find out to a hair how much they weigh." He added, "It is no unusual sight to see a dozen fat ladies in line at one of these machines waiting their turn. At the Windsor, American and other of the smaller hotels the same scenes are witnessed."[2]

After a reporter visited the cities of New York, Boston, and Washington, D. C., in 1884, he observed, "My recent visit to some of the noted watering places, and my observations of several large audiences since my return, has impressed me once more with the belief that the thinness and angularity of American women, so much commented on by Europeans in the past, is fast becoming traditional. They seem to be competing for fullness not to say stoutness, with their Old World sisters, who almost universally acquire an excess of flesh with the passage of their youth." He continued, "It is remarkable how few native women, out of girlhood, one meets nowadays in the large cities that have preserved their slenderness. Twenty years ago a round, plump figure was almost the exception. Now the exception seems to be the other way. The increasing avoirdupois of the daughters of the nation is too conspicuous to be ignored. It is probably due to the growth of wealth, and, therefore, of ease and luxurious habits in the community."[3]

That same year a man by the name of Professor Huxley declared that a full-grown man should weigh 154 pounds, of which 28 pounds was fat; 68 pounds was muscle; 34 pounds was skeleton; and three pounds was brain. Taking no account of height, for example, Huxley's idea of a normal weight was very crude but later in this period tables of "normal" weights based on height, gender, and much later bone density, would become fixtures on the American scene.[4]

Still in 1884, a journalist remarked that society women in Chicago "have been seized with a dread of obesity. The alarm is almost epidemic. The doctors have prescribed walking — at least thirty minutes daily. Fashion has decreed that the promenade shall take place between 4 and 5, and between those hours the avenues and boulevards are thronged with fat, rich ladies, from thirty-five to forty-five, dressed to their chins in furs and plush and resplendent in soft mufflers and gorgeous accessories." Those processions were said to include in their number "some of the wealthiest and best ladies in Chicago society."[5]

Also in 1884, a very brief news item declared, "Fat people are going out of style. Leanness is to be considered a mark of fine breeding."[6]

As the summer resort season reached its peak in 1885, at another area popular with the elite — Martha's Vineyard in Massachusetts — a reporter commented, "There are more fat women in this place than you can shake a stick at. Some of them tip the scales at 300 and 350 pounds. They come down here to get rid of some of their superfluous adipose, and for that purpose they bathe every day."[7]

An 1885 news story reported there was not much comfort for fat women as they contemplated the latest edicts of fashion because, "Fashion, for once, has completely ignored handsome, fleshy ladies, who look handsome because of their splendid proportions, although you never met one who did not tell you she sat up nights reading exhaustive treatises on how to become thin." The journalist worried the stout lady, in spite of her girth and ponderous walk, would soon be lost to sight to make room for the new creature of the hour, namely, the thin woman.[8]

A reporter writing in 1889 noted that in 1850 American literary icon William Makepeace Thackeray was writing about the York girl, and said, "The women here in New York, almost without exception, are as lean as greyhounds, and dress magnificently in the fashions of the better class of Parisian actresses." Then the reporter declared the likeness to the hound "has been lost in a single generation. American people are accumulating flesh, especially American women. Finding a woman who is passing the milestone of 35 and twice out of four times she is nervous about her weight and sensitive about her waist measure." Next he went on to mention the normal weight tables then in use by London, England, life insurance companies. They would not write a policy for any person five feet in height if that person weighed less than 98 pounds or more than 182 pounds. Those figures represented the minimum and maximum regarded as safe for that height. The average, or "normal" weight, based on data from the policies already written, was 115 pounds for that height. For a woman of average height, say 5' 4", the London rule was a minimum 119 pounds, maximum 161, with a normal weight of 140 pounds. A 6' tall man could not be insured if his weight was below 144 or above 196; normal was 170 pounds.

Roughly, the allowance made by the tables was about five additional pounds for every extra inch in height.[9]

On April 5, 1895, the Village Trustees of Jamaica, Long Island, directed the local outdoor advertising billposter to tear down posters about a New York dime museum. Those posters featured a "dozen stout women attired in tights, engaged in a bicycle race," and the offending advertisements were removed the next day. After the posters made their first appearance in the town about one month earlier, they generated much comment "and the question as to whether they were up to the Jamaica standard of morality was warmly discussed." A local interest was added to the subject when it became known that one of the bicycle riders was a resident of the village.[10]

Journalist Katherine Morton gave a table of weights for women in a 1906 article with the suggestion that any woman who weighed much over those figures should take steps to lose weight. Those figures were: 5'1" 120 pounds; 5'2" 126; 5'3" 133; 5'4" 136; 5'5" 142; 5'6" 146; 5'7" 149; 5'8" 155; 5'9" 162; 5'10" 169; 5'11" 174; 6' 178 pounds.[11]

According to a 1907 article, many out-of-town observers said the women of New York City were fond enough of food "to be on the high road to obesity." One visitor declared that he had been studying the women in a fashionable restaurant and "Every word that caught his ear had something to do with eating...it was all about cooking and what to eat, the variety of entrees to be found in famous restaurants at home and abroad..."[12]

Life insurance data also became the primary source for studies that looked at weight and mortality rates. One of the earliest of such studies was done by Dr. Brandeth Symonds in 1908. After studying the data of some 200,000 people he concluded that a person was better off being underweight than being overweight. Symonds found the lowest death rate did not coincide with the standard (or so-called normal) weight, but was found in the class of people that was about five percent below standard weight. At any age above 30, however, the ratio of actual deaths to expected deaths rose with the percentage increase of overweight. For example, a group of men 5'6" tall, each weighing 195 pounds, which was 30 percent above the standard, would have an actual mortality rate of 172, as against 100 expected deaths for the standard weight group. A long-lived ancestry did not reduce the excessive mortality of the overweight of 30 years and up although a short-lived ancestry exacerbated the mortality rate. Overweight foreigners were worse risks than the native-born obese. Symonds concluded that the person who was slightly underweight had a better chance of living than one of average weight and in all ages above 30, weight falling even as much as 20 percent below the insurance table's average did not appreciably increase the mortality rate.[13]

An article that appeared in newspapers in 1911 wondered why there were so many fat women. "I have watched the passing throng in several cities in this State during the present summer, and while one fat man was passing by I have counted not less than four fat women," he explained. "This ratio has held true whenever and wherever I have had occasion to take observations. These women are for the most part between 35 and 55 years of age. They either waddle ponderously or propel themselves forward with not the slightest perceptible freedom of motion, looking the while like statues being moved on rollers." He said he had observed them in large numbers at different summer resorts, both inland and on the Atlantic coast and that they ate with exceeding gusto. Continuing on he declared, "The alarming corpulence of our middle aged women is getting serious. They seem to be fattening for a slumberous old age. At one summer resort where I spent a week recently it was almost tragic to watch them seated on piazzas or in lounging chairs on the lawns, immovable as statues, patiently awaiting the hour for lunch or dinner, at which time they would arise and propel themselves slowly indoors, resembling nothing so much as a fleet of galleons in the eighteenth century."[14]

Mrs. John S. Flannery, president of the Housekeepers' Co-operative Association of Pittsburgh, launched a 1913 protest against fashions in that city's department stores. "What chance has a fat woman got with such styles? Slim and scrawny women have a monopoly," she complained. "Whoever started the theory that skin and bones constituted beauty anyway? This thing has gone on long enough and it has now got to stop." The women's editor of the New York *Tribune* agreed with Flannery and added, "Fat women in all cities should arise. Mrs. Flannery has sounded the clarion call. Let fat women everywhere respond. Disagreeing was the editor of the *Oakland Tribune* who observed, "a really fat woman has no chance with any style. If that be treason let the Heavy Brigade of Pittsburgh make the most of it."[15]

By this time there were many articles appearing in the press that advised fat women about the type of fashions they should buy in order to look less fat. For example, a 1915 advice column in the *Washington Post* advised its obese female readers not to wear a tight skirt, but a dress with a full skirt, and so on. "My experience of the fat woman is that she loves to sit at home, eat the best of everything, and then rely on an expensive quack medicine and her dressmaker to make her thin. My advice to her is very old — exercise...and let the medicine and, most of all, the dressmaker, be the last resort."[16]

Alfred Malsin was a mechanical engineer who brought science to clothing manufacture for stout women, or so he claimed in 1916. He said he applied the laws of physics, mathematics, optics, psychology, color, and so on to the design of clothing so stout women would not look so stout — in response to what he said were many, many complaints from fat women that they could not buy clothes off the rack that suited them. In an attempt to define the term, Malsin said, "The term stout, as I use it, means either a person who is not well proportioned, either bust or waist or hips being larger than the other two; or a person who is well proportioned, but whose body has reached a size above normal." Despite the problems with his definition Malsin went on to try and estimate how many stout women there were in America, a task few others, if any, had attempted to undertake. He said he studied census reports, received data on the body measurements of over 200,000 women from a life insurance company, and personally measured 4,500 stout women in department stores. At the time there were 33,049,399 women over 15 years of age in America. By Malsin's calculations 40 percent of that number, or 13,219,759 women, were stout — either stout all over or so stout in some one part of their body that their symmetry was destroyed. Of those 13,219,759 stout women, 5,685,438 were what he termed excessively stout — that is, they had busts measuring 44 inches or more. Thus, the excessively stout women made up 17 percent of America's female population over the age of 15, in 1916. That percentage varied according to age, steadily increasing from two percent for women aged 16 to 19, to 69 percent excessively stout for women aged 70 years and over.[17]

7

Psychology and Effects, 1920–1939

Dr. Leonard Hirshberg, a physician associated with Baltimore's Johns Hopkins University Medical School and a syndicated newspaper columnist writing on health topics, declared in a 1921 column, "Almost every sensible woman knows that she would be happier if she was slender.... Man, lazier, more comfortable, and less interested in his tropic of cancer, ignores his rotund porch front. Both, however, have one thing in common, to wit, a wish for some easier way, short cut or magic medicine that will 'do the trick' for them without effort, work, exertion or deprivation." And that explained why quackery with respect to obesity treatment never went away. Still, the period 1920 to 1939 was marked by the arrival of a much more scientific and logical approach to fatness. Calorie counts and weight tables were heavily used and relied upon. Less and less frequently did the medical community come up with silly ideas and notions regarding the causes of obesity. More and more the cause was acknowledged to be a very simple equation — that is, obesity was a function of calories in and calories out. Because it took time to become overweight and perhaps even more time to regain normal weight through the only effective method — adjusting calories in and calories out — the search for the magic bullet continued, as did quackery.[1]

Winifred Black wrote a newspaper column in 1922 that was in response to remarks made in Los Angeles a few days earlier when Dr. Lulu Hunt Peters of Los Angeles (herself a medical columnist) rose up in

116

a public meeting in that city and said "It is a disgrace to be fat." Black argued Peters had gone too far, "It certainly is a nuisance to be fat and it certainly is a bore to be fat and it is certainly ugly to be fat — but a disgrace! Isn't the fat itself enough of a punishment doctor — without your rushing out after us with such a bludgeon as 'disgrace?'"[2]

Called the "high priest" of feminine fashion in France, and one of the foremost dress designers, Paul Poiret gave a 1923 interview on women's figures in which he stated, "We do not pay much attention to fat women. They are the infirm among the fashionable. We cannot do anything special for them. They have merely to trail along the path of La Mode. Their case is not for the dress designer — it is for the physician." Reportedly, that was distressing news to obese women because up until then many of them had been consoling themselves that if they were not slender they could dress to appear so, but would be rendered disconsolate by the cruel statement from Poiret. "In their confidences with other women they had explained how a line here and a color there had made all the difference of 30 pounds on their figure," explained a reporter, "But Poiret has upset all that fine optimism, scathingly declaring that if you weigh 180 pounds you will look 180, and not 170." And, "To be sure, the fat woman can look neat and pleasing. But stylish and beautiful. Never, declared the French fashion designer." According to the reporter, books that dealt with the topic of how to become thin and how to stay thin would become even more popular and in demand as women tried to match the figure of the "scrawny flapper." Weighing scales were said to also be more popular with some of the scale manufacturers having said they had recently received orders to install scales in private homes so that female members of the family could weigh themselves before and after eating, with and without clothes.[3]

Poiret elaborated his point, saying that if the fat woman wants to be beautiful she had better get a reducing diet from a doctor and go to a masseuse. He added, "Many men will not go to the opera because, as they express it: 'They don't like to see a heavy meal sack of a woman tiptoeing onto the stage as though she were a dainty coquette.' For some reason or other opera singers are invariably fat. No doubt in developing their voice they have developed all parts of their bodies, which became more plump as the voice becomes fuller and richer." According to the reporter there were very few people in the world who thought the fatter a woman was the more beautiful she was. One exception was said to be the Turks, among whom fatness was prized as one of women's greatest charms. Explained the story, "the Turkish women can eat, and indeed are encouraged to eat, all of the bonbons and sweetmeats they want. They know no dietary laws except to eat only fattening foods. They sleep about fifteen hours a day in order to preserve their soft fleshiness and loll about on cushions and rugs the rest of the time." And, "Were an American woman to do this she would be considered a mountain of ugliness and be compared to the fat lady of the circus." Showman Flo Ziegfeld was said to have recently hired seven Turkish women — former members of the ex–Sultan's harem. Stating they were all very beautiful women when viewed through the eyes of a Turk, Ziegfeld admitted they would all have to go on a strenuous diet before he would let them appear before the public in the "Follies"— his theatrical revue.[4]

At that point the reporter moved away from Poiret for a moment and got bizarre when he claimed that cave men admired very fat women because, in the first place, when famine came cannibalism was practiced. Additionally, he claimed the modern infant of 1923 preferred a stout nurse. "Many people think that the men of the cave period went too far in the fat direction," he explained. "Some of the ladies were said to have weighed four hundred pounds and everything was done to keep them at this ideal weight." No evidence was presented in support of such fanciful ideas. Getting back to Poiret, the journalist said the Frenchman looked at the matter from the French point of view and threw up his hands at the fat woman. "You rarely see a fat woman in France, for the French, of all women, are desirous of being beautiful and to them that means being slim. The typical French beauty is slender and willowy almost to the point of scrawniness," said the American reporter. "In this country, where fat women are more common than in France, dress designers have not abandoned the problem of making the fat woman beautiful. They find ways of accentuating their good points and softening their bad ones by the application of scientific principles of color and line." Dr. Lulu Hunt Peters was said to have evidently taken sides with Poiret for she said, "It is a crime to be fat — a crime against love. Fat people are not lovable. To reduce in weight means to promote conjugal felicity." And, "It is natural but not necessary for women to add weight as they grow older. People should realize that after reaching maturity, which is about thirty years for both men and women, the body does not need food any longer for growth. It needs food only for upkeep and repair and energy." Peters agreed with Poiret that the only remedy for fat people in general was to study their diets or to consult with their physicians regarding their diet and to exercise daily.[5]

Fat men were also a subject of interest in France when the Goncourt Prize, one of the most coveted of France's literary awards, was given to Henri Beraud in 1922 for his novel *The Martyr of Obesity*, which had for its hero a very fat and very romantic Frenchman. Stirred up by the book was a debate as to whether or not excessive fatness was a handicap to a man in his love affairs. Several of the Paris newspapers invited their readers to say if they believed a woman was as likely to love a fat man as they were to love a man of normal size. Said Mlle. Parisys, the popular comic, "the stout man often is the friend of a woman, but he never becomes the man of her heart." Mlle. Therese Dorny, a well-known actress, said, "This discussion makes us women look at men as men look at us. As soon as they see us in their minds they disrobe us. We must either be pretty or shapely, else man is indifferent...In love stoutness plays a secondary role. I consider stout men awkward and discreet." Paulette Pay, a Russian refugee and actress, believed "a woman can easily fall in love with a stout man, on condition he possess a kind heart and shows devotion, which till now we had always sought in slender men." Madeline Cariser, a shareholder in the Mogador Theater wrote, "It is certain that a big stomach is physically displeasing, but, after all, to be able to eat well is surely some satisfaction. And then the stout probably become philosophers sooner than the others, and that is no mean advantage, but I, nevertheless, prefer the slim."[6]

Marcelle Carpentier, wife of the playwright, observed, "All the stout men I know have charming wives. I prefer the stout because they usually have frank faces, clear skin and happy dispositions. Because they are strong they are gentle; because they are gentle they are polite, and because they are polite they are good." William Johnston, a New York editor and novelist who weighed 250 pounds said, "I like to be fat" and to prove it he had written a book explaining how much fun he had in being a fat man. "High time for some fat man who is satisfied with his lot, who gets heaps of fun out of being fat, to come to the front for the fat," he explained. "So let me say, with all the weight of my 250 pounds — I like being fat. I am fat because I prefer to be fat." Johnston argued that any fat man could get thin if he wanted to and, "fat isn't a matter of food or exercise at all.

It's a matter of philosophy. Fat people are merely those who have learned to get the most out of life, who have discovered the things that are really worth while." And, added Johnston, "the fat man invariably enjoys a good reputation. He is the last person to be suspected of crimes or misdemeanors or any wrong doing." Also claimed was that fat men and women had a greater facility than did thin people in making and holding friends. "Fat men and women are popular because they are inclined to be liberal — liberal in their thoughts, liberal in their opinions, liberal with their time, liberal with their money, liberal in regard to other people's shortcomings."[7]

Mildred Holland was a newspaper columnist who tried to point out the advantages of stoutness in a 1923 article. Women active in business and the professions, she argued, invariably learned from experience the command of the average person's attention that was produced by mere physical bulk. "If that bulk is carried and dressed in a way which is awkward or even ludicrous, the attention it compels is of course of the wrong sort," she explained. "But garbed tastefully and poised with an effect of self-confidence and good balance, a goodly allowance of pounds is a real asset. It creates for the owner a certain sense of personal importance and invariably causes her to be noticed and remembered...In short, generous size is a personality advertisement." Another advantage Holland found was that the woman of middle age or older who carried excess pounds had the good-looks advantage in every way over her underweight sisters of the same size. "Curves are far more universally becoming than angles after youth is past," said Holland. "Young or old, the stout girl or woman can invariably make herself an attractive and individual type."[8]

Living in Miami, Florida, in 1927, and depressed over a steady gain in weight, Mrs. Rebecca Levy, 31, a native of Russia, scribbled a note to her husband saying she was "too fat to live," and then ended her life by suicide in January of that year by opening the burners on her gas stove in the kitchen. According to physicians she weighed 180 pounds and was said to have brooded over the rapid manner in which she was gaining weight.[9]

Also in 1927, a news story from Toledo, Ohio, reported that fat girls were to be excluded from a $50,000 home for young women to be built in that city 50 years into the future through provisions made in the will of David Bourdette Burgert, bachelor and member of one of Toledo's oldest families, who died on February 8, 1927. The will provided for the erection of a home with the luxuries and conveniences of its time for "women

120

between the ages of 16 and 28, of small stature (no fat women need apply), bright, ambitious, stylish and good to look at. It is between these ages that youth yearns for better things in life and it is this kind that I here provide for." It was to be a residence for women with a love for beautiful things that parents could not provide. Burgert's estate was to be placed in trust for 50 years (with the income going to David's two sisters). At the end of that period the funds for the building of the home, to be known as the Burt Burgert Apartments, was to be provided.[10]

Over in Switzerland the Cantonal Tribunal of St. Gall tried a strange case in April 1927 when a tradesman asked that judicial body for a divorce from his wife — described as a "huge woman"— on the sole ground of "abnormal obesity." The husband's petition declared the wife ate as much as four people and his savings were squandered in buying food for her. She was said to have taken a dozen different medicines in an effort to reduce her appetite and her weight but without any effect. After due deliberation the amused jury dismissed the petition, declaring that obesity was no cause for divorce.[11]

Putnam, Connecticut, was the location of the death of 64-year-old Henry Appleby who committed suicide on August 29, 1933, by hurling himself down a well on his farm in Putnam. Appleby weighed over 350 pounds and according to Dr. S. Overlock, the medical examiner, had become increasingly despondent because of his obesity.[12]

According to a story excerpted in 1920 from a publication called *The Modern Hospital* a discerning, but unnamed, hospital superintendent had discovered he needed fat men at the information desk and on the switchboard of his institution, to help make things run smoothly. Some time earlier, the superintendent explained, he determined to find the cause for the rather constant criticism of his institution; criticism he felt to be wholly unwarranted since he was certain that the medical work, the nursing and the food and service were all excellent. But, in spite of that, there seemed to be a tendency among the public for uncomplimentary observation that was difficult to analyze because the criticisms were vague. By a process of elimination the superintendent determined the trouble was at the very entrance to the hospital, at the information desk. "The quick, nervous types that I had at the switchboard and the entrance I had thought very efficient. I suppose I thought so because they were quick, but I was wrong," he explained. "They didn't stand the strain well, they did not lend themselves to the other man's point of view. To them a visitor was an intruder. And now I'm going to have a big good-natured man, two if necessary, men who will wear well, who can smile, and who will make people good-natured in spite of themselves. It takes a fat man to do that."[13]

Subscribing to the idea that laziness was one of the prominent traits of fat people was Charlotte Beehler, swimming instructor at the Baltimore YWCA. Observing her class of fat women swimming at the YWCA in 1922 she commented, "Why do women wait until they look like frights before they start to reduce?..It's because they're mentally and physically lazy — the fat women, I mean." Charlotte said she had 50 fat women in her class, 20 of them weighing over 200 pounds each and "only one woman is seriously working to reduce her waistline. She really works in the pool, and I never feel that the moment my back is turned she is floating leisurely and comfortably." Beehler fumed that she wished some of those fat women's husbands could see them "working" in the pool, "I'd like to tell those husbands the truth! The truth is they work hard about ten minutes, not longer, and then float and talk. Oh, how they love to talk!" Several of the women had made it a practice to bring a bag of cakes down to the pool to eat between laps, "And up in the cafeteria after the swimming lesson, you should see them gorge. They hate to have any of the physical instructors come into the cafeteria and look at their trays!" Beehler's advice to fat women was; "Don't wait until you're as big as a house and look like a fright before you start reducing! And take it seriously. Some women reach 200 and then come here and expect to shake off fifty pounds just floating and talking." She spoke of a hike she and one of the other instructors had taken the fat women on the previous spring, "It wasn't a very long or difficult hike, but they insisted upon having their chauffeurs follow after us so when they got tired they could be picked up and taken home."[14]

James C. Young wrote a 1923 article about the honesty of fat men, declaring that his statement was not a philosophical conclusion but, rather, a fact established by the man who underwrote the insurance industry's policies. According to their records there were fewer fat men found to be embezzlers than any other class of people. "They simply could not [embezzle]. There is too much kindliness and sunshine behind their smile. They are the sort that sleep o' nights. To put it another way, fat men are lethargic and less stirred by the passions of life," enthused Young. "They think slowly and act slowly, and men who reason and move that way are less inclined to hear the call of the Circes than those who are impetuous. Thus fat men have better judgment all around than their more ardent brothers, especially when it is a case of personal welfare — of their very destiny." According to Young these surety firms that insured against theft and embezzlement preferred to issue a bond for a man with a 44-inch waist than for a thin one. "They believe that the perspective of the fat man is several shades happier than that of his fellows, and by so much he is regarded as a more favorable risk." Young argued that the man who happened to be both fat and profane was an even better risk, that is, a safer bet. And the thin man given to cursing was a better risk than the silent, brooding type. It was not the swearing per se, that made such a man a safer bet, but the emotional safety valve cursing provided. "Just as the fat man is a better risk than the thin man, and the man who is both fat and profane rises in the scale of honesty, so the fat and profane man of middle age is the best risk of all. By that time he has got rid of any lingering passions likely to lead him astray."[15]

A little over one year later Fred M. Withey, vice president of the National Surety Company of New York, told members of the Columbus, Ohio, Advertising Club that men with hobbies and fat men usually were good risks for surety companies. The man with a hobby was said to be too busy with his pet subject to take other people's money and the fat man "is a good risk because his thoughts center on eating rather than dishonesty." As well, the married man was a better risk than the bachelor by a margin of six to one. Withey also noted the violently profane man was a good risk because he took out his peeves in swearing rather than in stealing. Women, as a rule, he added, were more honest in business affairs than men. And when women did go wrong, he said, "their speculations usually are not large."[16]

Three years after that, in 1927, Harry Huff, an actuary with the National Surety Company, declared he had statistics to show that fat men were a more honest lot than were thin ones. A news story remarked that the firm praised the honesty of other large classes, "women, the married in general, Chinese. But it has a special word for the stout."[17]

Still later, in 1931, Dr. Kinzo Saza of Japan asserted that "Fat men are honest." Reportedly he had "proved" that idea in a thesis submitted to the Imperial University at Kukuoka, Japan. He was awarded an honorary degree for his research. Saza's investigation covered the life careers of thousands of criminals. He found that very few fat men ever committed criminal acts and those that did could be easily reformed. Most criminals were said to be slender and to have been so all their lives.[18]

Experiments designed to study conditions as they might affect miners were conducted in a specially constructed chamber in 1924 at Pittsburgh by the United States Bureau of Mines. One finding from those studies was that fat men stood the heat better than did thin ones. The fat men, the bureau found, lost more weight when subjected to uncomfortably hot temperatures, but they were less exhausted when they were relieved.[19]

Dr. Neil A. Dayton of the Massachusetts education department conducted a study of 3,553 retarded children in the public schools of Massachusetts, in 1921 and 1922. He found the average intelligence of children who were above average in height was seven points higher than the average of children who were under the normal height. Children who were overweight had an average intelligence six points above those who were underweight. When children were both underweight and under height the difference in intelligence scores was even more marked.[20]

In Atlantic City, at a 1935 session of the American and Canadian Medical Associations, Dr. Walter R. Campbell of Toronto asserted that the use of too many carbohydrates in the diets of unemployed people as an economy measure might convert many of the 25 million people then on North American relief roles into permanent unemployables since they tended to put on fat and become lazy. Campbell said that for the American continent unemployed peoples' diets were tending to be high in carbohydrates because diets high in protein and fats were relatively expensive. "Excessive carbohydrate often leads to obesity when given to people without work to use up the energy supplied. Carbohydrate eaters are often distinguished by fatness and physical and mental apathy," he explained. For those reasons Campbell suggested that the "apparently inevitable degradation from unemployed to unemployable should not be accelerated by a falsely economical provision of foodstuffs."

8

Oddities, Sports, Clubs, Employment, 1920–1939

Mrs. George A. Kenna, known in circus side shows for years as "Trilly the Fat Lady," died early in 1922. She quit the circus some 16 years earlier and made her home in Chicago. When she died she weighed 400 pounds and while she was with the circus her weight was said to have exceeded 500 pounds. By this period the fat people in freak shows were largely a thing of the past. Dime museums had long since been swept away by the overwhelming popularity of vaudeville. While fat ladies could still be seen in carnival sideshows they were nowhere near as numerous as in the past and those that still existed were much less prominent and attracted little or no media attention.[1]

A new system of taxation was said to be ready, in early 1923, to be introduced shortly in several cities of Sweden. Under that system citizens of both sexes would have to pay a tax for every pound they weighed above 200 pounds. Authorities in those cities said they saw no other way of raising the money to pay for needed civic improvements. Citizens were said to be clamoring for new pavements, new sewers, new waterworks, new parks, and so on. In the opinion of the tax experts, every class of citizens was paying as heavy a tax burden as could justly be placed on its shoulders, with one exception — fat people. In the city of Gutenberg when citizens came to the city treasurer's office to pay their usual taxes, when the new system was implemented, they would be weighed and a tax imposed for each pound over 200. Those weighing 250 or more would have to pay a surtax in addition to the regular tax on their excess flesh and for those who reached the 300-pound mark, there was still another surtax. Of course, the fat people in Sweden were up in arms and promised to carry the matter to the highest court in the land. The following reasons were given as to why it was alright to tax fat people more heavily than normal-sized people; "Fat citizens, dragging their ponderous weight about, subject sidewalks, pavements, bridges and other city property to a great deal more wear and tear. They consume more of the city's drinking water. Their bulk often constitutes a serious obstruction to traffic in busy streets. They break down the benches in the parks and the chairs in museums, libraries and other public places." As well, it was argued they were, by virtue of their size, the least active of any citizens in promoting the city's welfare; they tended to make other citizens slow down due to their own moderate rate of moving about and working and "their continued complaints about the heat and other things that cause them discomfort often make them little better than a public nuisance. They pay only one fare on the municipal motor buses and street railways, but occupy two and sometimes three seats. They mar the aesthetic aspect of a city and give visitors a bad impression."[2]

Along the same lines was a proposal that was made in Berlin, Germany, in late 1935 when the radical anti–Semitic weekly *Judenkenter* suggested what was needed was the introduction of a special tax on obesity on the ground, "pot bellies are superfluous and superannuated in the new Germany." The proposed tax would depend on a person's girth, the paper said, with steeper amounts fixed by authorities for every centimeter over a certain limit. Exemptions would be permitted only if obesity was the result of a malady or if a person could prove that reducing his weight would injure his health. Jews would pay an extra amount, an even higher belly tax because, said the publication, "statistics proved the standard of living of German Jews was 17 times higher than that of Aryans." Thus, the belly tax on Jews would be 17 times higher than the one levied on Aryans.[3]

Fat men's races at picnics, field days, and so on, continued to be held in this period, but to a greatly diminished extent. Such events had likely disappeared almost completely by the time of World War II. At Ossining, New York in September 1922, John Sancarato, 305 pounds, won the fat men's race at Sing Sing Prison's annual field day games, inside the prison walls.[4]

The Washington, D. C., Board of Trade's annual shad bake was held in May 1923 at Chesapeake Beach, Maryland. Some 800 men made the trip to the event, which featured various athletic events. One of which was the fat man's race, won by Frank Parsons who weighed around 240 pounds.[5]

In June 1930, more than 500 alumni, representing 30 classes, held the first alumni day in the history of the City College of New York. Most of the afternoon was devoted to a field day, which consisted of many athletic events for the alumni. A prize for corpulence was awarded to Samuel Jacobson, class of 1922.[6]

A reporter commented in a 1921 article that it was then a common saying that a fat man could not play golf. Such a man "is thought to be ashamed even to try...Outright obesity is regarded as an anomaly or a fatal disqualification on the links," according to the piece. Yet, the reporter declared, golf was proclaimed as a cure for stoutness, which meant that some fat men must have played the game and reduced. In England, supposedly, the matter had been studied scientifically and it was found that of 10 men over the age of 80 who played golf regularly not one was stout — nine were lean or reasonably so while the tenth man was "moderately stout." A cynic might object, added the journalist, that one almost never saw a fat man over 80 whether a golfer or not. But, reportedly, six of the 10 80-year-old golfers had been stout at 50 and "It was the game that had brought down their weight and relieved them of uncomfortable embonpoint. The physiological reasons for this are duly given. Swinging golf clubs opens the chest and gives the oxygen a chance to burn up the material which otherwise would be laid down as fat. Thus the unhealthy stout man grows leaner on the links."[7]

Among the cabin passengers who sailed in December 1922 for Rio de Janeiro and Buenos Aires on the liner Vasari was Miss Margaret Hoffer of Richmond Hill, New York, who weighed 348 pounds. She was on her way to Montevideo, Uruguay, to give an exhibition in swimming and diving. She had won a total of 14 medals, including three for high diving. When she went to her cabin on the ship she found it was impossible to get into her berth. A carpenter was called in who made two berths into one and placed stanchions underneath. Hoffer had to keep her trunk in another cabin, and dress there as well.[8]

Fat men's clubs that existed purely as a social organization with little purpose other than to offer members one or more special, gargantuan meals over the course of a year also continued to exist, but also to a greatly diminished degree. At a horse show in New York City in November 1922, a special feature was a luncheon given by Alfred B. Maclay president of the National Horse Show Association in honor of what had been known as the Fat Men's Club. A condition for membership had been that the applicant had to weigh a minimum of 275 pounds.[9]

About one year later some 250 men of average weight and 150 fat men gathered in the ballroom of the Hotel McAlpin in New York City at the Fat Men's Luncheon of the Rotary Club. Before the luncheon there was a hotly fought weighing contest. Winner was restaurant proprietor John L. Manna, who tipped the scales at slightly over 300 pounds. In a prominent place in the ballroom was a huge placard describing a fat man's favorite menu. Dishes included clam chowder, fish cakes, tenderloin steak and onions, mince pie and cheese, with chocolate and whipped cream; the calories from that single meal were listed on the menu board as 3,161.[10]

At the start of 1931 president Carl Shaw of the United States Fat Men's Club announced that the financial depression resulting from the 1929 stock market crash had reduced the bulk of his club's membership by around 3,650 pounds, leaving the gross avoirdupois of the association's remaining 1,472 members at a total of 332,672 pounds (an average of 226 pounds per member). Thus, the club was campaigning then to attract new members.[11]

Employment effects of obesity continued to center mainly on police forces. An official report on the physical condition of Atlanta, Georgia, policemen was made in 1932 by city physicians. In the aggregate the police force, numbering 322 men, was described as being 3.5 tons overweight (an average of 21 pounds of excess flesh per officer). Almost one-third of the men were too fat, about 25 percent had poor eyesight and bad teeth, 50 had flat feet, 26 could not hear as well as they should, 30 suffered from kidney disease, 21 had heart disease, and two were "mentally deficient." According to a news story, "Too much fat and too little muscle appeared to be the major complaints found by the examiners." Those examining doctors recommended to Atlanta Police Chief T. O. Sturdivant that every overweight officer be placed on a diet and compelled to take half an hour of physical exercise every day. The diet recommended included oyster stews, fresh fish, chicken broth, boiled or poached eggs, cheese, clam broth, beef tea, graham and gluten bread and zwieback biscuits. Beverages were limited to water, buttermilk, tea, coffee, and mineral water.[12]

New York City Police Commissioner Lewis J. Valentine expressed a preference in 1938 for young, agile rookies with college training and experience in group athletics. He deplored the fact that many applicants then being appointed to the force were 33 or 34 year sold, some of who were getting "bald and corpulent."[13]

The "evils" of obesity figured prominently in advice given in March 1939 by New York City Mayor Fiorello La Guardia and Police Commissioner Valentine to 20 young women and 23 young men who were being sworn in as probationary officers in a ceremony at police headquarters. Although they were warned by both city officials of many and varied types of pitfalls ahead in their careers on the force, the new members were instructed particularly not to use elevators where they could climb stairs, to watch their diet and to take plenty of exercise to keep themselves physically fit. Valentine warned the new officers, "We don't want to see you taking on weight too rapidly — or at all. If you do you won't be half as valuable to the department." In referring to Valentine's remarks, the Mayor declared the day of "the round-helmeted, handlebar-mustached, fat policeman was over." However, La Guardia admitted he was not sure how a person could prevent himself from becoming fat.[14]

Besides police running afoul of weight standards, one overweight teacher in New York City created a great deal of controversy in the mid 1930s and caused the board of examiners of the city's schools to issue its opinion that teachers who were overweight were not "acceptable hygienic models" for their pupils and did not stand the strain of teaching. Miss Rose Freistater, 30 pounds overweight according to the board's standards thought otherwise and had carried to the State Commission of Education her fight to obtain a regular license as a teacher. The board of examiners, in support of its refusal to recommend a license for Rose, forwarded to the Commissioner a brief setting forth its views on the relationship of weight to teaching. Although there had been a number of cases of overweight or underweight teachers before the board since the standards were set up 10 years earlier, Rose was the first to appeal to the State on those grounds. Her appeal was sent to the Commissioner of Education in May 1935. Since Rose was first refused a regular license in 1931, she had taught 277 school days at James Monroe High School as a teacher-in-training and a substitute teacher. Her department head had commended the excellence of her work. But she was still 30 pounds too heavy for her 5'2" of height, by the board's standards, and so could not obtain her license as a regular teacher unless the State Commissioner overruled the board. Freistater was 26 years old. Actuarial standards for the teachers' pension system were said to have had much to do with the board's refusal to recommend a regular license. Substitute teachers were not members of the pension plan but regular teachers were, and had to be, members.[15]

The board of examiners argued it would not be fair to members of the retirement system to admit people not fulfilling minimum requirements, and it would not be fair to the children to license teachers who could be subject to ill health or physical disabilities, such as heart disease to which obese persons were subject. Rose replied that she felt her four years of experience showed she was able to take the strain. After her appeal was filed Rose was examined again, on June 26, 1935. She still weighed 180 pounds. In 1931 she weighed 182. The maximum allowed by the board for her height was 150 pounds with 120 pounds regarded as "normal." Back in 1931 she had been given six months to get her weight down, in accordance with custom. She lost 20 pounds during that period and asked for an extension of time to lose the rest. However, the board refused to grant her an extension. The board of examiners told the Commissioner that medical experience indicated that markedly underweight or markedly overweight persons had relatively higher mortality and morbidity rates than person of normal weight, especially in middle life. "Other things being equal, a person of abnormal weight is therefore likely to have more frequent absences because of ill health and be less efficient as a teacher than a person of average weight," argued the board. "The reduced expectancy of life of such persons would moreover, tend to constitute a drain on the pension fund." According to a reporter, very few applicants for a teaching license had ever been refused because of their weight. Most people not in compliance with the standard initially were able to reduce or gain sufficiently in the six-month period of grace. After a teaching license was granted, observed the journalist, the education authorities made no further checks and that meant licensed teachers could gain, or lose, as much weight as they pleased.[16]

The issue of Rose's weight was controversial and publicized enough to generate an editorial in the *Washington Post*. "On the surface the controversy over Miss Freistater's weight appears a little absurd and not without humor. In the face of her training and ability to perform the job which she has selected as a vocation, it seems ridiculous that she has been weighed and found unwanted," said the editor. "But there is a much more serious aspect to the whole question. Are teachers in the public schools of New York to be selected for their fitness as instructors or because they are good retirement risks?"[17]

A month later the case was still pending with Rose represented by a lawyer by the name of Arthur Mabel, who declared that Rose gave "no appearance of excessive stoutness." Rose explained to him she had been trying to reduce her weight by horseback riding, hiking, and tennis at Ithaca, New York, where she was enrolled in a field course at the Cornell University Summer School. However, her weight reportedly remained at 180 pounds. "She's a sturdy, solidly built girl and it would be dangerous for her to reduce," added Mabel. The board continued to oppose Rose's application for a license arguing a teacher of her weight did not have the necessary fitness to perform the work, "Teachers must climb stairs, take part in fire drills and be able to handle all real school emergencies. Overweight teachers are less likely to stand the strain of teaching."[18]

On December 11, 1935, Rose and her lawyer appeared in Albany, New York, before the State Education Department at a public appeal granted to Rose in her appeal from the license denial. They explained that Rose's weight was down to 154 pounds, fully dressed, and that therefore she was entitled to her license as a permanent teacher since her weight was now at least "close enough." The board of examiners, however, remained opposed as she was still over the maximum weight, albeit by only a few pounds. A few months later, in early 1936, the state denied Freistater's appeal on the ground she had been too late when she filed it, thus she was denied her permanent teaching certificate.[19]

9

Causes and Effects, 1920–1939

The attribution of obesity to silly and strange causes and reasons had almost completely disappeared from the scene by this time period, at least when such attributions came from respectable members of the medical and scientific communities. Dr. Leonard Hirshberg observed in 1921 that obesity was more than a lack of comeliness and grace; that overweight often carried various penalties such as high blood pressure, diabetes, heart disorders, cramped lungs such as Caruso's pleurisy, a crowded condition of the internal structures in the chest and the abdomen, obliterated arteries, fallen arches, arteriosclerosis, appendicitis, and constipation. Adipose tissue, he said, "999 times in the 1,000 implies too much food or too little exertion, or both." In other words, he emphasized, a person must work hard or play hard every day and "eat a simple, country fare of leafy fruits and vegetables, yeast, dairy products and as little meat as you need." He added that there was no "natural" physiological gain in weight after the age of 40, as a lot of medical books then still taught. "If you gain in fat and are unconcerned about it, you are like the business man whose expenses are greater than his sales. You are accumulating a dangerous liability. It will be the cause of ruin and disaster." Hirshberg regarded fat as a millstone that would carry its bearer to an earlier than expected grave but that a person could become lean "by avoidance of the life of the well-to-do, who are exposed to too much good food too often, who have an excess of comfort, no money worries and a plentiful supply of ease."[1]

A decade later Dr. Alonzo Taylor asserted, "Overeating, relative to need, is the major cause of overweight." He remarked that the daily muscular work being done by the average American was declining every year, the result of the mechanization of society. As well, the automobile had greatly reduced the average annual amount of walking done by people. Extreme hard work required a daily intake of 6,000 to 8,000 calories, he said; hard work 4,000 to 5,000, light work 3,000 to 4,000, sedentary occupations required less than 3,000 calories per day. In Taylor's opinion the easiest way to avoid overeating was to consume bulky foodstuffs with low calorie content instead of concentrated foodstuffs with high caloric content and "It is in this respect that fruits and vegetables are attractive; they are invaluable for vitamins and mineral elements, but they are also valuable in satisfying hunger and appetite without promoting overweight." With the national income rising and the proportion going to food declining, Taylor said it meant the possibility of overeating was increasing, "Unless restrained, a decade hence the average overweight of people over 40 will be significantly higher than it is today; the effect of overweight upon incidence of disease and upon the death rate will become more conspicuous."[2]

One of the few bizarre attribution came in 1934 from Dr. Ramsdell Gurney of the University of Buffalo medical department. Gurney argued that stoutness in human beings was inherited according to a predictable law. One hundred cases, all women, were studied in the outpatient department of the Buffalo General Hospital. Only 20 percent of the children of stout parents were found to be thin; only 10 percent of the children of thin parents were found to be stout, while the offspring of a stout and a thin parent were found to be about evenly divided between the two conditions. Gurney went on to point out there was no subject on which there was so much disagreement as that of obesity. While that conclusion was perhaps valid at an earlier time, 1880s to 1890s, say, it was not true when Gurney did his research.[3]

Physician Logan Clendening remarked in 1937 that in the treatment of obesity it was becoming more and more the idea that simply cutting down food intake was all that was necessary. But, "The overweight often refuse to accept this, especially the implications as to cause. Most of them say they do not eat as much as other people — that some mysterious process inside the body operates to keep some people fat and others thin."

Clendening felt that such false hypothesis could be grouped into three types: 1) anomalies of metabolism, 2) unusual conditions of the endocrine glands, or 3) peculiarities of the nervous system."[4]

One of the most bizarre of the attributions came in 1938 from Doctors Mark F. Lesses and Abraham Myerson of the Boston State Hospital's division of psychiatric research. Writing in the *New England Journal of Medicine* they argued obesity could be the result of mere mood, saying, "People who are restless because their lives are unsatisfied may be seen nibbling candy, nuts, crackers and the like." They declared there was a technical term for that way of becoming obese, and that term was "anhedonic obesity" (anhedonic is the absence of joy in doing things that bring joy to normal persons). Anhedonics could be put through the usual paces to reduce their weight — exercise and diet — but what was the good since it was the mood that had to be reached. It also happened, while doing their research, that Myerson discovered the remarkable effect of benzidrine sulphate "in cheering up lunatics who were ready to commit suicide in a fit of depression." Lesses and Myerson experimented with 17 fat patients, all were described as "nervous nibblers." Their sense of well being increased after benzidrine sulphate was administered; they were less interested in food and more in the affairs of the outer world. Since less food was eaten, their fat melted away. "With mildly nervous patients the drug is just as effective when obesity follows ordinary overeating or lack of exercise. The best results are obtained when the diet is low in calories. When the patients are so neurotic that benzidrine will not elevate their moods the treatment is useless."[5]

Ida Jean Kain was a lay columnist who often wrote on health topics such as obesity. In a 1938 column she urged her readers to limit their intake of salt, sugar, snacks, and water, and observed the average American used five to ten times as much sugar per day as did the average person abroad. Kain discussed the role of water in obesity as that liquid — so long and wrongly blamed for obesity — was slowly rehabilitated to the harmless and blameless zero-calorie liquid that it was. "The average overweight person drinks too much water with meals and too little between meals," said Kain. "Water cannot make you fat, but it does increase the appetite. Taken at the beginning of the meal water stimulates the appetite, too much with the meal stretches the stomach, and taken at the end of the meal water remains in the stomach, thereby stretching it further and increasing the food capacity." Kain added that if a person was serious about losing weight that person would restrict the total liquids taken with meals to eight ounces, "This little dietary rule can make an amazing difference on the scales. Drink all the water you wish between meals. It does not influence your weight."[6]

Six months later Kain mentioned in another one of her columns the work of Pittsburgh physician Dr. Frank A. Evans, said to be a leading authority on obesity. Evans argued that obesity was the result of overeating, not something glandular, and so on. And that while many overweight people insisted they did not eat much, no more than people of normal weight, Evans said that was not true.[7]

In 1939 Dr. Logan Clendening stated in one of his columns that it was remarkable how many theories had been advanced to explain obesity, "remarkable considering that in 98 per cent of all cases the cause is simply consumption of too much food."[8]

This period marked the first time that articles on obesity could be found that dealt exclusively with the diseases and health effects that came from being fat. Diseases were, of course, mentioned in earlier times but almost always as part of a more general article in the subject. By this period, though, the bad health effects of obesity were discussed more frequently, seriously, and more in-depth. A 1921 article asked its readers if they weighed more then than they did at the age of 30. If so, said an editorial writer in the *Journal of the American Medical Association*, you were too fat. Because the age of 30 marked the period of full maturity and the proportions that were normal then should be maintained through life, declared the editorial. Life insurance experts then considered the possessor of excess fat to be liable to all sorts of ills, with diabetes being one of the chief such ills. Physicians had long noted the liability of the upper class to diabetes, and the greater propensity of that class to be overweight. "The increment of body weight is so commonly observed, particularly among the well-to-do classes, toward middle life that it is often looked on as a natural or physiologic gain which is to be expected after the age of forty," said the editorial. "As a rule it causes little concern to those who are thus adding to their size, unless the gains are of sufficient magnitude to produce discomfort in certain types of activity or to occasion disfigurement from the standpoint of prevailing views on the human physique." On the basis of statistical data, life insurance firms had long insisted that being overweight was a physiological liability rather than an asset. Those who maintained the proportions of the age of 30 (assuming normalcy) exhibited the most favorable mortality. As to the burdens of obesity, the editorial said, "Tissue fat must be carried about like any other incubus. We are reminded that overweight puts a strain on the heart and on the joints, and that it pushes up the diaphragm and cramps the lungs." A vicious cycle was soon established because "The obese person inevitably limits his exercise; he grows heavier from the unused reserves, and his activity thereupon becomes even more restrained and limited. Overfeeding, obesity, and lack of exercise interplay until 'big' becomes 'bigger.'" According to the medical journal's editor, diabetes was largely a penalty of obesity, and the greater the obesity, the more likely was nature to enforce it, "There is a wide-spread tendency on the part of many clinicians to explain — perhaps one should say excuse — obesity as the result of constitutional causes independent of mere overeating in ultimate analysis...diabetes as a sequel to infectious diseases may be an expression of the overfeeding of convalescence."[9]

Writing in 1923, Doctor W. A. Evans declared that the largest single factor in high blood pressure was obesity and that was the conclusion drawn by the Life Extension Institute after it examined the data from over 16,000 policyholders of the Metropolitan Life Insurance Company. It was found that policyholders that were 30 percent or more above the best weight for their age had an incidence of 16 percent with high blood pressure, more than 20 percent higher than the expected number. Of the so-called normal weight policyholders, only six percent had high blood pressure. According to the story, obesity as an attendant of high blood pressure did not come into evidence until after age 25 and it reached its maximum at the ages of 45 to 55. After age 55 lean people were almost as likely to have high blood pressure as overweight people. Noting it was difficult to decide what factors were involved in high blood pressure Evans declared, of the Life Extension report, "Nevertheless, the information helps. The indictment of the fat man is valuable because it is one of several. Nearly every grand jury that sits on his case votes a true bill."[10]

At an address made in Chicago on August 25 Albert M. Johnson, president of the National Life Insurance Company, before a convention of insurance men, declared that obesity "is killing off Americans at such a rate that the special education of those afflicted with excessive fat is needed." Without giving specific details Johnson went on to say that it was more dangerous to be fat than it was to travel on an ocean liner, ride on a railroad train or "tempt fate in an airplane."[11]

In one of his 1925 columns, physician Dr. W. A. Evans observed there was a saying, "Nobody loves a fat man," before going on to mention Dr. Dubray who had long studied the problem. Dubray declared, "Obesity is one of our most common diseases." He observed there were many diseases associated with obesity such as diabetes, high blood pressure, and other forms of heart, blood vessel and kidney disease. "The obese are very liable to have gallstones and other gall bladder troubles. This applies especially to fat women. Fat women are very prone to amenorrhoea. Many of them have dysmenorrhea. Fat people are more than average susceptible to rheumatism. The cancer rate among fat people is higher than among thin ones. Fat people do not stand operations well," said Dubray. As well, he added, the average life span was relatively short in fat people with the people who lived to a ripe old age generally being "the hard, slim, spare, lean, dry kind." Dubray pointed out that the weights given in the height/weight tables and generally thought of as being the "proper" weights were only average weights, "They are not best weights. The best weights for people over 30 years of age are 10 to 20 percent lower than the average weights. The people about 15 percent below the average weight are the best risks, according to the insurance companies.[12]

A report from Dr. Louis Bauman, director of the metabolism ward at Presbyterian Hospital (New York City), determined that of the last 215 patients requiring operations for gallstones at Presbyterian Hospital, 88 percent were overweight.[13]

An editorial writer declared in a 1931 editorial in the *Journal of the American Medical Association*, "Fatness in persons over thirty-five is now generally considered risky, if not positively dangerous." According to the piece, widespread interest in the manifestations of overweight, or obesity, in man belonged to comparatively modern times. A German clinician, the late Professor Ebstein, once grouped fat people into three categories; those who inspired envy, those who occasioned laughter, and those who called forth sympathy. An American colleague added that fashions in America were such in 1931 that the first group no longer existed. "There have, of course, always been instances in which discomforts of undue bodily size awakened concern on the part of the obese and promoted measures for suitable relief," said the editor. "A more serious attitude has been developed in recent years by the publication of statistics gathered by life insurance actuaries indicating an apparent penalty for overweight." And, said the medical publication, there was the problem of disease. "The apparent relation of diabetes to obesity is another feature that has brought overweight within the realm of thought of many persons," declared the editor. "In the presence of wasting disease or of undernutrition, diabetes is practically unknown. Persons who habitually overeat are especially prone to diabetes...The warning has been broadcast widely. It seems to be substantiated by much statistical evidence." A hopeful sign for the editor was the inroad made on national overweight that was due to the fact that among women at least, it was then stylish to be thin. As to the cause of fatness, the editor said the attempts to relegate obesity into the category of specific disease were then meeting with little favor, "The storage of fat appears to be primarily a feature of metabolic bookkeeping — an indication of the favorable balance between energy intake and the actual requirement of food fuel." In conclusion, the editor stated, "Living conditions of the present day have been conducive to the reduction of muscular work and exposure. Appetite has not declined accordingly; nor has the ready availability of food in a day of higher standards of living. The outcome is one that must be faced frankly."[14]

A brief news item in 1939 said it was estimated that about one out of every three people who had diabetes was overweight.[15]

10

Reducing, Diets, and Exercise, 1920–1939

Obesity was a large enough issue in the 1920 to 1939 period that its control and treatment became a public health issue, in many communities. For the first time efforts to have people lose weight moved out of the hands of the medical community and the quacks, and came to encompass society in general. One of the first such efforts took place in Chicago. On April 22, 1920, 20 females volunteers who weighed on average 220.5 pounds began a six-week officially sponsored course in reducing under the direction of the city Health Commissioner John Dill Robertson. For the following six weeks home gardening, long walks, prescribed diets, and "accepted" reducing exercises would comprise their program Robertson had initially called for 50 volunteers, half men and half women but only 20 fat women and one fat man answered the call. When he found himself alone the fat man fled the scene. The women were to don overalls on the following day and take an hour's exercise in their respective backyard gardens, with spading, hoeing, and weed pulling included in Robertson's instructions to them. Twelve of the women were housewives, two were typists, one was a stenographer, two were clerks, one was a buyer, one was an office manager, and one was a nurse. On a daily basis the women had to telephone Dr. Robertson for advice on exercise and diet and each Thursday the entire group met with Robertson in order to be weighed.[1]

Two weeks later it was reported there were a total of 24 women in the eight-week program and that the course was for severely fat women.

Two weeks into the program there was said to be an average net loss of 8.3 pounds per person. At the end of week one there was a loss of 3.9 pounds, and at the end of week two a loss of another 4.4 pounds. Leading the way at the time was Mrs. Hilda Solberg who had lost the most weight, dropping from 224 to 212 pounds in the two weeks.[2]

Those 24 women who were aged from 20 to 49 with a weight range of 166 to 231 pounds (plus one at 323 pounds) had an average starting weight reported in this piece as 201.5 pounds. All the women were more than 40 pounds over a normal weight. Much publicity was devoted to the story with the campaign slated to run for 60 days and with all the women having agreed to stick to the regimen for the full 60 days, including a pledge to stay on the diet prescribed by Robertson. The doctor commented the program would have plenty of outdoor work and "As bending and stooping are necessary, there will be work over the wash-tub and the similar household devices. All manner of exercise will be ordered." As well, the exercises would be adapted to the particular case as some of the women were engaged in vigorous employment and some were not. Diets would be "severe," Robertson warned, but would also be tailored to the individual case. Generally, though, starchy foods, breads, cereals, butter, cream, potatoes, and so on, were on the banned list while salads, spinach, cabbage, Brussels sprouts, fish, and lean meats were the types of foods the doctor had recommended. In general, said Dr. Robertson, "As a people we are too obese. We are stall-fed. If we had lived like the Indians, had each day taken all manner of violent exercises, even if, like them, unconsciously, we would have no stout persons except, perhaps, those whom sickness or old age prevented from active life."[3]

By far the most publicized of all such public health initiatives that took place was the one in New York City. On October 18, 1921, it mobilized 50 fat men and 50 fat women into a reducing squad with a reported, and grandiose, goal of losing an aggregate of 5,000 pounds by the middle of November when New York City Health Commissioner Doctor Royal S. Copeland planned to present the 100 "heavyweights" at the city's health exposition as an example of what stout persons could do in the way of becoming more becoming. All the participants were told to start in on the program with their breakfast meal on October 19. Then the plump women were to get into bloomers and middy blouses for the first daily workout in the gymnasium at Madison Square Garden. Among the heaviest of the participants was a 5'6" man who weighed nearly 300 pounds and a 5'2" woman who tipped the scales at 274 pounds.[4]

While the above report appeared the day before the program began it was premature in that no men participated in the program, only 50 fat women. And on the 19th those women in bloomers struggled for an hour on the roof of Madison Square Garden to do bending at the waist exercises and other gyrations, under the direction of "Philadelphia Jack" O'Brien, officially the athletic instructor of the women's division of the fat reducing team that was training to win prizes at the Health Convention slated to be held in November in Grand Central Palace. Copeland, director of the project, said he believed there would be desertions by the participants before the month ended. He also said he was surprised at the number of men and women in New York City who wanted to reduce their weight. Since the fat-reducing contest was announced he had received hundreds of letters from people wanting to get thin. Many letters from women urged Copeland to form night classes, for people who were not free in the daytime, when the program took place. On October 19, 12 unregistered women showed up at Madison Square Garden on their own initiative, in an unsuccessful effort to join the group. Their names were placed on a waiting list that would be used to fill vacancies left by deserters. Official menu for the program for October 19 was as follows: Breakfast — choice of orange juice, or prunes stewed in lemon juice; any of the standard cereals, with a tablespoon of bran sprinkled over it and with skimmed milk, but no sugar; one coddled egg on dry toast; tea, coffee, or skimmed mill with milk in the tea or coffee if desired, but no sugar. Luncheon — vegetable soup; two bran muffins, no butter; stewed spinach or lettuce salad, with vinegar or lemon juice for dressing, no oil; two or three slices of boiled tongue (avoid the fat part); apricots, no sugar; tea, coffee, or buttermilk. Dinner — clear meat broth (grease removed); hot or cold lean roast beef (do not eat any fat), celery; boiled onions; two medium slices of whole wheat bread; fruit gelatin (use any fruit except bananas); tea or coffee clear; plenty of water between meals, very little salt on food, and one tablespoonful of petroleum (mineral) oil upon retiring.[5]

As early as October 20, just two days into the program trainer Jack O'Brien reported that some of his charges were already showing a loss of flesh. Reductions were also confirmed by reports that reached the Health Department. One woman was reported to have dropped 10 pounds, going from 208 down to 198 pounds while a second participant had decreased from 180 to 175 pounds. Some waistlines had dropped by from one to three inches. A hike by the group was scheduled for the following Sunday but specific plans were not made public as O'Brien did not want the route known, with a lot of spectators perhaps turning out to have a look at the 50 fat women.[6]

Five days into training one of the participants told O'Brien that she had that morning laced her own shoes for the first time in several years while another said she had picked up a fallen glove without calling for help from a family member. From letters received by city health officials there was evidence that hundreds of women, and men too, were following the diet prescribed for the 50 participants — it was available in a hand-out version to the general public as well as being published almost daily in the newspapers. Also, discussion had developed as to whether Dr. Copeland had not been too liberal in the diet prescribed. Some held that prunes had no place on the bill of fare and others contended there were too many eggs. Even some of the participants were among those who felt the Commissioner had been overly liberal and announced they intended to cut out lunch during the remainder of the month-long program. That day's menu was as follows: Breakfast — juice of an orange or whole orange; two bran muffins; cereal, any of various kinds, with a tablespoonful of bran sprinkled over top, skimmed milk if desired, but no sugar; tea, coffee or skimmed milk; skimmed milk could be taken in tea or coffee. Luncheon — clam broth or vegetable soup with the vegetables left in; two medium slices of whole wheat bread; sardine and lettuce salad (two sardines); whites of two eggs coddled on one of the slices of whole wheat bread; celery; tea, coffee, or buttermilk; skimmed milk in tea or coffee if desired; stewed prunes (no sugar in cooking them or consuming them). Dinner — four raw oysters with lemon juice or cocktail sauce; two bran muffins; baked halibut basted with tomato sauce; spinach or cauliflower; fruit gelatin (any fruit but bananas); tea, coffee (black); a tablespoonful of petroleum oil upon retiring; plenty of water between meals.[7]

When O'Brien questioned his group the next day he said the loss of weight averaged from two to four pounds. Every woman involved in the program agreed that diet and exercise were great for producing sleep. Besides the 50 officially in the program the 12 reserves had been carrying on a course of unofficial training. The 62 obese women gathered at Madison

Square Garden daily at 10 A.M. for exercises first on the first Sunday of the program and then were to set out on a hike in Central Park (the route was revealed to the public in the end) with the length of the hike to be "the limits of endurance" of the fat women.[8]

When the hike was held Fifth Avenue was crowded with a Sunday throng when the women marched along it to Central Park, "attracting attention at every step, being followed most of the route by interested spectators," said a reporter. Entering the park at 59th Street the squad went over most of the main paths and then back to their quarters at Madison Square Garden for another session of calisthenics. While in the park some of the women tried to add the exercise of tree climbing to the hike. "The police frowned on this and shunted the climbers back to the path," it was reported. Some of the women lounging in the park got up from their benches and joined in the hike with the result "There were more than 100 women following the squad as a rear guard when it returned to Fifth Avenue.[9]

When the first week of the program ended O'Brien revealed that the average loss of weight for the squad of 50 was six pounds and five ounces. However, two of the women recorded a weight gain, of 2.5 and 1.5 pounds, respectively. According to a reporter, Copeland said, "the fat women had entered more into the spirit of the thing and they were not simply driving themselves through unwelcome exercise in order to get thin, but that, so far as he could see, each one of the women now enjoyed the training and found it interesting."[10]

A news account of October 27 said that policewomen in plain clothes were shadowing the 50 fat women. Learning that several of the participants, hungry under the diet prescribed, had broken training to eat more bread than permitted or consumed pancakes and syrup, instead of lettuce and celery, Health Commissioner Copeland issued a warning. Addressing the group after their calisthenics he said, "I am watching you. I have interested the plain clothes men and they are following you around. Each day I get a report and I know the ones who are cheating. You must stop that."[11]

Two of the participants had confessed to Copeland that they had broken training. At the same time he was warning his dieters he defended his diet against the criticism that it was too liberal. "To my mind, one great trouble about all these methods of reducing is that the patients are starved to death. They go around looking half starved. They have a wild look in their eyes," explained Copeland. "There are certain things which you could take into your stomachs which do not make fat. That might be said of sawdust, but I wouldn't recommend that. Things like celery and lettuce do not make fat. They don't make much of anything, but they fill the stomach. I don't want anybody to go to bed hungry." At the start of the program 27 of the women weighed over 200 pounds, with the heaviest at 281. Smallest were two women, each of whom weighed 150 pounds, to start with. That day's menu was as follows: Breakfast — apple sauce (no sugar); any fresh fruit except bananas; dry toast made from any kind of bread; cereal, any of the varieties, with one tablespoonful of bran sprinkled over the cereal, skimmed milk, no sugar; coffee or tea, no sugar, skimmed milk in the tea or coffee, if desired. Luncheon — clear beef broth, with grease skimmed off; vegetable salad, vinegar or lemon juice, no oil; two slices of bread at least 24 hours old; celery, all you want; tea, coffee or skimmed milk. Dinner — roast chicken, no dressing, do not eat the skin; spinach, all you want, vinegar or lemon juice; sliced tomatoes, very little salt; two bran muffins, no butter; fruit jelly, any kind of fruit except bananas; tea or coffee clear, no sugar. One tablespoonful of petroleum oil before retiring, plenty of water between meals; limit the amount of salt used.[12]

So much interest was aroused by the project that Copeland could not begin to answer all the questions posed in the letters he had received from the general public as so many letters had been received. In investigating why one of his participants had gained weight he discovered she had supplemented her training by taking a whole box of obesity pills. Some of the participants asked Copeland to let them eat figs and dates but he refused. A prize was to be awarded to the woman who lost the most weight (since the starting weight of the participants ranged from 150 to 281 pounds a fairer way would have been to award the prize to the woman with the greatest percentage weight loss — instead of absolute poundage lost). Sarah Mell, who had been near the top of that list, fell several places in the standing when her weight went up about two pounds overnight — she confessed to Mrs. Elsie Thompson, the supervising nurse, that she succumbed to temptation and had eaten a pound of nuts one night. After 10 days of the program Sarah Strong led the way with a loss of 16.5 pounds — she started at 281 pounds. Copeland continued to defend his diet, noting a good many still criticized the diet as having too much food included. He said that careful study of his diet would show that while the quantity seemed larger than one involved in reducing should consume, the menu was made up of proteins, and proteins did not make fat. "This reducing squad is causing much interest. One of the most frequent questions is whether the women will put on weight after the month of diet and exercise. If they go back to former living habits they surely will," Copeland said.[13]

As of October 28 it was said that Copeland feared a possible revolt as some of his 50 fat women had threatened dire things if the last line of the daily menu — "One tablespoonful of petroleum oil before retiring" was not eliminated. Apparently they disliked the taste of the oil. However, it was not removed from the menu, remaining a part of each day's bill of fare, with no further protests about the oil publicly recorded. Copeland's latest advice to his participants, and to thousands more who unofficially followed the menus was to avoid certain foods and obesity medicine. "Starches such as you get in bread are fattening. I understand that some of you are taking medicine for obesity. You must not take medicine. Medicine taken in connection with these exercises and diets is likely to do you harm," he explained. Also, he advised people to drink coffee and tea without sugar and if they could not do without a sweetener, then to use saccharine.[14]

On October 29, Copeland estimated that the 50 obese women under his supervision had dropped approximately eight feet of their total waistline in 11 days. Mrs. Jean Dwyer reported her waist had dropped six inches from the start. Copeland had received many letters asking him to establish a diet kitchen where those who wanted to reduce could get not only food to meet their requirements but also "expert advice" on how to grow thin. His response to such suggestions was, "I am not in the fat-reducing business. But it must be a profitable one."[15]

In the words of an October 30 news story, since the fat program began, "the interest taken in their training and diet has been tremendous." Letters to Copeland poured in from every part of the country. Not only did those letters come from ordinary citizens who wanted treatment but also from doctors and health officials in many places inquiring as to the diet and the method employed in conducting a fat-reducing contest. As well, some 500 requests for night reduction classes came from fat women who could not find time for training during the day. It was reported that a girl of 12 wrote for help, who was 50 pounds overweight and "Girls from fourteen to seventeen years of age and weighing from 165 to 250 pounds write." (This is probably the earliest reference — anecdotal and un-quantified as it was — to fat children). The writers of some of the letters seemed to think the Health Commissioner had discovered some secret for reducing weight. But he disclaimed having any knowledge other than the secret of proper exercise and diet. "It is safe to say that every popular magazine has asked for a special article on fat reducing. I have had letters from nearly every State asking for details and an endless number of afflicted women have telephoned for permission to join the class," explained Copeland. "There is no doubt that as a spectacular undertaking it is a great success. Our purpose was to attract attention to the Health Exposition in Grand Central Palace in November, but incidentally it has revealed that thousands in our city are honestly anxious to get rid of superfluous flesh." He went on to say the program had demonstrated several interesting things. One thing was that hunger was satisfied in a wrong way by very many people, "When the stomach is empty it communicates with the brain and a call for food is sounded. Likely a drink of water would satisfy this yearning but instead of taking water a quantity of chocolate candy, or ice cream, half a pound of sweet grapes, a handful of raisins, dates, figs or other similar articles is taken. These but add to the fat fuel."[16]

As far as Copeland was concerned the greatest mistake people made was in the selection of their food with the average meal being poorly balanced. That, he said, was particularly so of breakfast, decrying a typical morning meal of cereal and cream, hot muffins with butter and honey, sausages, and possibly some fruit covered with sugar. It was an entire meal — made up of starches and sugar, which added to flesh. Copeland argued there was no secret in a system of fat reduction and that no system could succeed unless the candidate for leanness had taught herself food values and was willing to stick to a plan until the goal was reached. He thought it was easier to say what foods ought not to be eaten than to set down those that were safe to take. However, he said certain food could be consumed "abundantly," with some of them being celery, buttermilk, radishes, endive, lettuce, tomatoes, watercress, clams, whites of eggs, chicken without the skin, shad, white meat of lobster, codfish, pears, apples, grapefruit, lemons, oranges, rhubarb, lean meat, and skim milk. "Don't forget in reducing flesh exercise is important. One cannot expect to get thin when all the exercise taken in a day consists principally of getting on and off cars. Let me repeat again that all these things may be done with good result, but if a person goes back to the old method of eating it will all have been done in vain," he emphasized.[17]

On October 30, the second Sunday of the program, the 50 fat women were taken on a long hike in Central Park and afterward put through more strenuous exercises than on the first Sunday, at their quarters in Madison Square Garden. Physicians agreed with their trainer O'Brien that the two weeks' work had hardened and strengthened the contestants so that they could undertake a more severe course of calisthenics and outdoor exercises. By that time, said Copeland, over 400 women had applied to him for permission to join the group. Most of those women had no interest in prizes, but were anxious to reduce and better their health. To those women Copeland said it would not be convenient for the New York City Health Department to continue any further efforts of that sort of supervision after the current program reached its end, "but I will be glad to assist any interested groups of women who may desire to take up similar work. We will provide them with the data, together with the rules for indoor and outdoor exercises, and the details for proper dieting, and with this it will be easy for any body of women to proceed intelligently. If they keep at the work faithfully they will find that it is comparatively easy to overcome excess fat, brought on by years of over-eating and lack of exercise."[18]

After two weeks of the program the total weight loss of the 50 women stood at 482 pounds. Sarah Strong continued to lead the way with the largest weight loss — 21 pounds. Second place was held by Mrs. Ella Weaver (19.5 pounds). The day's menu was: Breakfast — apple sauce, flavored with cinnamon, no sugar; choice of any cereal, bran sprinkled over, skimmed milk may be used, no sugar; the whites of two eggs on toast, no butter, tea, coffee, no sugar, but may add hot milk. Luncheon — one cup of clear broth; fruit salad consisting of orange, apple, celery and lettuce, no sugar or oil, the juice of the orange is sufficient; two bran muffins, no butter; tea, coffee, no sugar, buttermilk. Dinner — strained tomato soup or clam broth, no milk; small piece of broiled steak; green string beans; cucumber with salt and pepper, vinegar but no oil (use very little salt); celery; two rusks; clear gelatin; tea, coffee, no sugar, very little skimmed milk. And, as always, one tablespoonful of mineral oil to be taken before retiring every night.[19]

In his quest for information on the effects of his diet and exercise program on the fat women Copeland questioned the husbands of some of the women and found they all experienced great relief— a relief that increased with every pound that their wives lost. Said one husband, "Taking the wife out for a walk used to be an ordeal. Now it is a pleasure." Another said it was an unwritten law in his family that whenever his wife went upstairs he should assist her ascent by pushing from the rear. But he no longer needed to do that. Yet another husband reported he had to do most of the family washing in the past but now rejoiced because his wife could bend over the laundry tubs.[20]

Three weeks into the program it was reported that 39 participants had survived to that point. The ten with the greatest absolute weight loss were to be the guests of the Public Health Exposition to be held in Grand Central Palace with the one having lost the most weight to receive a prize from Copeland. One of the participants said, "I don't care whether I win a prize or not but I feel better and look better and I am more active. Just how much may be set down to imagination. I cannot say, but the way I get up stairs reminds me of ten years ago, when I was classed as young."[21]

On November 12, 1921, the remaining 35 women in the fat-reducing contest were weighed for the last time as the Health Exposition started the following day. Winner of the prize for losing the most weight (31 pounds) was Sarah Strong, 32, 5'7" tall, who weighed 281 pounds at the start and 250 pounds at the program's conclusion. Her measurements at the start of the contest, and at the end were, respectively, 52", 50", 60", (47.5", 39", 53"). Second place went to 33-year-old 5'8" Ella Weaver who lost 28.5 pounds, an average of 16.5 pounds was shed by the 35 finishers.[22]

When the Public Health Exposition at the Grand Central Palace was closed on the evening of November 19, with the presentation of various prizes, New York City Mayor Hylan presented Sarah Strong, winner of the fat reduction contest, with a silver cup.[23]

Two months later, on January 17, 1922, there was a reunion at the Health Department Building in New York City of most of the fat women who started their reduction program on October 18 and finished it on November 14. Fifty women had started, 35 finished the program, and 20 showed up for the reunion. But, said a news account, "they are still fat." Copeland asked those in attendance how many had gained weight since the class ended; six hands were raised. How many had lost weight, he queried; up went eight hands but three wavered and then went down.

When he asked how many weighed more than they did when training began, no hands were raised. During Copeland's discussion with the group there was a sudden crash when the leg of a chair broke letting 249-pound Ethel Gray crash to the floor. She weighed 270 pounds at the start of the program. Of contest winner Sarah Strong, all that was said was, "She has put on some weight since November."[24]

As of October 14, 1922, 600 new applicants (with an average weight of 200 pounds each) had been admitted to the Fat People's League, enlisted in the fight to elect Dr. Royal S. Copeland to the United States Senate on the Democratic ticket, in that year's election, according to Georgia Heffner, president of the League. Membership of the group was made up of men and women whom Copeland as Health Commission had helped to reduce. In order to qualify for memberships men had to weigh 180 pounds or more; women had to weigh 160 pounds or more. Heffner said she was personally heavily indebted to the candidate for relieving her of 80 pounds of superfluous weight — by following the heavily publicized program's diet and exercises. Originally Heffner tipped the scales at 240 pounds.[25]

Copeland was elected United States Senator and was next heard from in October 1925, when it was reported the former health commissioner of New York City would enter upon yet another new role shortly, that of restaurateur. That became known when, a day earlier, the Royal S. Copeland Restaurants, Inc., was incorporated in Albany, New York. Senator Copeland said his new firm would confine its activities to teaching people how and what to eat. "The idea grew out of a magazine story I wrote recently, in which I said that people learn how to do everything except how to eat and how to choose their foods," explained Copeland. "Some well-to-do friends of mine challenged this view and said that they had plenty of money to back the experiment if I was willing to run restaurants in which people could have an opportunity to learn the right kind of foods to eat." He added, in other words, we plan to conduct a series of restaurants in which thin people can get food to give them proper nourishment and fat people the kind of food to make them thin. It was the company's hope to begin with three or four outlets and to open the first two in the coming month or two.[26]

In Washington, D. C., female employees of the veterans' bureau reportedly had started a new fad in 1923 in an effort to lose weight — during the noon hour they climbed the stairs in the 11-story building that housed their agency. Many women were said to be involved in the unofficial program with the originator of the idea unknown but rumored to weigh more than 200 pounds. Although the fad was then largely spontaneous and unorganized it was speculated that the formation of a formal club with contests, prizes awarded, and so on, would soon result.[27]

According to a 1924 news account, the application of "common sense" to reducing had been tried lately in the home office of the Metropolitan Life Insurance Company and it was said to have shown good results. A survey done by the firm of their employees one year earlier had revealed 550 persons each of who was 20 or more pounds overweight. Of those, about 150 had so far taken advantage of the weight loss program run by the company. Said Dr. Haynes H. Fellows, physician in charge of the program, "The reason for our success is that the method is easy, harmless and slow." Only a small percentage of recruits to the program dropped out before completion and that, said Fellows, "is due to the simplicity of the diet requirements and the fact that the patient can include anything in his or her diet, allowing for it on the daily allowance." (This was a step forward in that there was no such thing in this diet as "dangerous" foods.) The reporter remarked the combination of exercise and regulation of the number of calories consumed was not new. "Most people have trouble in figuring out the caloric value of a given dish," explained Fellows. "We have developed a table of foods which contain one hundred calories. For instance, two small baking powder biscuits, three pieces of zwieback, one cup of oatmeal, one tablespoonful of olive oil, one large banana, one large orange, one-half a cup of stewed rhubarb — all these contain one hundred calories. After a little practice our patients become expert in determining off hand the caloric value of a given dish. This simplification is our chief contribution." Fellows went on to note that each person in the firm's weight reduction program was allowed a certain number of calories a day, figured on the basis of his or her proper weight. The formula called for between 16 and 20 calories per pound, depending on the type of work and activity during a day. If a person weighed 150 pounds, his daily caloric allowance would range between 2,500 and 3,000 calories. (This was one of the earliest reducing plans that made calorie counting and number of calories consumed a centerpiece of the plan. That is, the dieting aspect of weight loss was put on a much more scientific, and accurate, basis than at any time in the past.)[28]

With respect to exercises, Fellows explained that in his program they prescribed only 10 a day, of one-minute duration each, mostly bending and stretching ones, "These exercises mainly effect the hips and abdomen where the need is greatest and which the patient is most likely to neglect. Here again simplicity is the keynote." He said many of his successfully reduced patients had stopped coming to him regularly but kept him informed and that none had regained any appreciable amount of weight because, "The habit of correct eating once formed is just as difficult to break as the habit of overeating." Since figuring the caloric value of a given meal was a difficult thing for most people, the program that Fellows oversaw furnished all those in the plan with a booklet containing a list of the majority of foods reduced to the standard of one hundred calories. For example, an ordinary slice of bread, a "fair-minded" pat of butter, a piece of beefsteak .75 of an inch thick and measuring 2.0 inches by 1.5 inches were each 100 calories. "It requires little ingenuity for a reasonably intelligent person to become accurate at estimating a meal," said Fellows. "Our reducers furnish us the valuation of their meals weekly. The records are filling out our lists so that when we issue a new booklet we will have a complete list of nearly every sort of dish."[29]

Seven years later, in 1931, a follow-up report on the Fellows experiment was given; that overweight reduction class for the employees at the home office of Metropolitan Life Insurance Company had a total of 294 men and women involved in it. Treatment consisted, said the account, almost entirely of dietary restriction, with some exercise. Patients were interviewed once a week. After a period of supervision lasting from a few weeks to several months, according to the individual, 81 percent of the class had lost weight, with the average loss being 15 pounds. About 14 percent of the group lost as much as 30 pounds each. Those participants were followed up for five years after their treatment was completed. At the end of five years 21 percent of the patients showed a further loss of weight; this group lost an average of 10 pounds during treatment and nine pounds in the ensuring period. But once medical supervision was removed, there was considerable slippage. At the end of the first year there were 224 of the original group available for examination, only 32 percent had continued to lose weight and the majority had gained. Whereas they had lost an average of 17 pounds during treatment, they regained an average of nearly 10 pounds during the following year. At the end of the fifth year, said Louis

Dublin insurance executive, the "great majority" had more than regained what they had lost. He concluded, "They lacked the self-control necessary to continue the required abstinence. Apparently medical supervision is essential if good results are to be maintained."[30]

At a 1924 meeting of the American Medical Association Dr. Solomon Strouse told an audience of physicians, with respect to the obese, "When they eat fat it does not act as fats do in others. Certain effects from eating lean meats and eggs are not the same in the obese as in normal people." However, Strouse did not elaborate. Also discussing the topic of obesity at that meeting was Dr. McLester, who strongly advised against the use of thyroid extract as a reducing medicine. He recommended obese people to use a diet that allowed for a weight loss of from 0.5 to 1.5 pounds a week and that exercise should be mild and of long duration rather than violent. In particular he advocated cold baths for all who reacted well after them because "A cold bath causes the body to burn up large amounts of fuel." McLester urged that fat be eliminated nearly entirely from the diet as "the obese do not need it and if it is eaten the results are not what a normal person expects to get from fat." That meant the almost total elimination from the diet of butter, gravy, lard, cream, fat meats, and all other greases. He advocated a diet for people that gave a small quantity of foods, consisting of a fair amount of meat, a moderate amount of starch and sugar, and plenty of green and watery vegetables, and no fat.[31]

A lengthy 1925 article in the *New York Times* discussed what it saw as a growing fad of fat women trying to lose weight, "reducing has become every woman's concern." And, "Some merely toy with the practice. Perhaps they tip the scales at 130 pounds. They would much prefer to read 125 and they shrink from 140; and so they listen when others propound favorite reducing recipes. They return from card parties determined to subsist on raw cabbage and buttermilk — excepting parties, of course. They are strict with themselves for a week, then they weaken. Still they forego potatoes and call it reducing." Others listened with strained attention when the convention turned to the relative merits of milk and potatoes or pineapple and lamb chop. When the woman attempting to lose weight could no longer bear the gibes at home from the daily weighing on the bathroom scales many women resorted to weighing themselves away from home. The restrooms of department stores were said to be the best places, "Pennies drop into the slot all day; and the air is heavy with sighs." Sometimes they weighed themselves a second time, hoping for a different result, or weighed themselves from store to store, "All a store needs to do to get women's trade, say the cynical, is to train their scales politely to lie."[32]

With respect to the obesity remedies then available the 1925 *New York Times* article remarked, "there are rolling pins that massage the muscles four ways at once and just roll off the fat." Reducing girdles were said to have become almost the feminine uniform. Such items were popular, thought the piece, because at first it seemed easier to wear something than to give up eating, but soon the overweight woman returned to seek the latest in reducing literature, and there was always plenty of that. Turkish bath managers told people to sweat out their fat while a swimming instructor passed out the magic word and soon had a pool full of adherents. Said a dancing teacher, "I'm just swamped with middle-aged classes. They'll go through anything to reduce and call for more...Reducing ardor goes to such lengths that when they have finished the regular course they supply themselves with a little phonograph, a set of scales and a book of lessons. Then they dance more or less as their gains or losses suggest and the written instructions direct." Among others who were said to have benefited financially from the desire to reduce were the manufacturers of reducing phonograph records, and the distributors of "thinning" foods. Advertising people went out of their way to dissociate the wares they represented from fat, otherwise they could not hold a woman's attention, "The effect is just what he wishes if he can convey the suggestion that this or that will help her reduce." Candy manufacturers were disturbed when they heard that customers were counting calories, but the advertising man came to the rescue. "Thus car cards have come to recommend certain kinds of candy that 'satisfy the craving for sweet without adding an iota of fat.' Still, chocolate remained and chocolate is fattening. Even that, though, fails to stump the advertising man. This is his solution; 'Take a chocolate before every meal, reduce your appetite and watch your weight drop.'"[33]

Early in 1926 an announcement was made that a course of instruction in the prevention and cure of obesity would be given at the Columbia Heights Community Center in Washington, D. C., by Dr. L. F. Kebler, professor at Georgetown Medical School. The course was to include class work, diet lists, measurements and weighings. As well, there were to be elective co-related gymnasium exercises taught by Martha Dunham, a physical training instructor. Kebler was to tell of weight reduction by rolling, girdles, mineral baths, chewing gum, and the removal of harmful thyroids. He would also explain how overweight affected the heart, kidneys, and digestive organs.[34]

Newspaper columnist Viola Paris declared in 1927 that many women wrote to her asking her what they could do about their fat. She told them "sensible dieting" was the first step to the desired end. "As you already know, I am sure, potatoes, bread, meats, fat fish, pastries and sweets, and water taken with meals, all help to add that extra pound or two," she explained to her readers. "Fresh fruits, especially of the citrus variety and excluding bananas, dates, figs and prunes, all fresh vegetables, especially greens, and skim milk may be taken in moderate quantity." A typical menu from her was as follows, on arising — glass of hot water with lemon juice. Breakfast — was to be sliced oranges and two thin slices of dry whole-wheat toast. If desired, one boiled egg without butter. Luncheon — vegetable soup or some clear soup. Tomato and lettuce salad dressed with lemon juice; one raw apple. Dinner — a small portion of lean meat or fish; two vegetables such as spinach and cauliflower; a slice of bran bread, and raw celery, fruit salad with thin French dressing. All foods were to be cooked without sugar. Paris concluded her column with a lengthy series of exercises for reducing specific parts of the body, such as thighs, hips, and so on.[35]

Barnard College, New York, held its fourth annual health week in Brooks Hall in December 1927. At one of its exhibits the 1,200 students of Barnard were told what to eat to maintain a proper weight. A normal girl, they explained, required a daily intake of from 2,200 to 2,800 calories, according to charts of correct eating habits as prepared by the school's Department of Physical Education, led by Professor Agnes R. Wayman. Their recommended ideal daily diet was as follows: Breakfast — one orange (six ounces); oatmeal (one ounce) three tablespoons of cream, one teaspoon of sugar, one egg (two ounces); two slices of whole wheat bread (two ounces), one part of butter; one glass of milk (half a pint); total calories being 770. Luncheon — cream soup (one cup); peas (two ounces); macaroni, three tablespoons; lettuce (one ounce); one tomato (four ounces), French dressing; two slices of whole wheat bread (two ounces), one pat of butter; one glass of milk (half a pint); ice cream (three tablespoons); total calories, 1,060. Dinner — cream soup (one cup); roast beef, one slice (four ounces); carrots (two ounces); baked potato (three ounces); spinach (four ounces); lettuce (two ounces). French dressing; two slices of whole wheat bread (two ounces), one pat of butter; one glass of milk (half a pint); one-half grapefruit, small; total calories being 735. For the three meals the total calories were 2,565. For girls who were overweight the Barnard program recommended a "safe reduction diet" that reduced by 33 percent the normal maintenance diet of 2,200 to 2,800 calories, as follows: Breakfast — orange or grapefruit; one egg; one slice of whole wheat bread and butter; one glass of water. Luncheon — one large helping of freshly cooked fresh vegetables; one lettuce salad, French dressing; one piece of raw fruit (such as apple, pear, grapes); one slice of whole wheat bread and butter; one glass of milk. Dinner — two fresh vegetables; salad; one slice of whole wheat bread and butter; fruit; one glass of milk. Causes of corpulence were said to be, by the Barnard exhibit, "an inherited tendency to need less than the normal amount of food, sedentary habits of life and the wrong kind of food." Corpulence it was declared, burdened the circulation, causing palpitations, faintness, and high blood pressure. It also burdened the liver and the kidneys, broke down the arches of the feet and prevented proper exercise.[36]

Dr. Frank A. Evans of Pittsburgh, at a meeting in connection with a 1928 session of the Congress of American Physicians and Surgeons, said, "Obesity, which is increasing rapidly among Americans as a result of improper diet, can be remedied quickly by a radical dietary treatment in which the patient is given only from six to eight calories per kilogram of body weight as compared with 30 calories in the normal diet." More than 2,000 physicians from all over the U.S. attended the meeting. Evans asserted that weight reduction of as much as 100 pounds had been noted in patients given the new treatment. Since it was a diet that had to be carefully balanced and to contain an adequate supply of proteins and carbohydrates it meant a physician's supervision. That is, it was not a diet for a patient to take alone and unsupervised.[37]

A 1928 report from Dr. Louis Bauman, director of the metabolism ward at Presbyterian Hospital in New York City revealed that in the treatment of patients greatly overweight the average weight reduction was 15 pounds, for 183 patients. "The women patients far outnumber the men, due, apparently to the fact that women place a greater importance on their physical appearance," said the report.[38]

Washington Post columnist Viola Paris received so many letters from her readers asking advice on weight reduction that she addressed the subject in three consecutive columns. "Correct living, and particularly the habits of diet, are the fundamental principles. Exercise has its part, and an important part, but unwise eating or drinking may very well undo all the good work that exercise has done," said Paris. As well, she advised her readers to omit potatoes from their diet, consume raw fruit, except bananas, figs and prunes.[39]

In her second column in the series, Paris explained, "The person who is carrying excess poundage almost always has a tendency toward foods that are fat-building, as well as a tendency toward indolence that makes any sort of vigorous exercise far more of a chore that what it should be — a pleasure." She advocated outdoor exercise with swimming and tennis being especially commended and, "Every one should spend at least an hour each day at some exercise in the open air, if it is nothing more than a brief walk."[40]

During 1934 at a department store in downtown Washington, D. C., a corset "expert" (a representative of a corset firm) gave lectures at 11 A.M. and 2 P.M. for women on how to lose weight. According to a reporter, the expert did not just solely mention the benefits of her company's corsets — although she did that — but also mentioned other aspects of reducing, such as various diet plans.[41]

That same year in New York City, Arthur E. Bagley had a one-hour radio exercise program running daily except Sunday from 6:45 A.M. to 7:45 A.M. on station WEAF and six associated stations. He read the exercises out over the air and his listeners did them. At that time he had been doing the program for nine years and his show was said to be then the oldest continuous daily feature on American radio. The story had circulated that Bagley sat in a comfortable chair while leading the exercises. Said Bagley, "No. But I do not take the exercises; in fact no one does in the studio. I stand at the microphone because it is not possible to be enthusiastic about the work if I should sit down. So I stand there and read the instructions which take me about five hours each day to prepare." Over those nine years Bagley said he had received more than two million letters. As a result of audience requests he had distributed 2.1 million exercise charts and about 2.0 million pieces of health literature; pamphlets on overweight, underweight, prevention of the common cold, and so on. As of 1934, he had eight assistants employed to take care of the daily mail.

"The chief worry of most Americans seems to be overweight. I guess they believe in the theory that nobody loves a fat man," added the radio personality. "It is estimated that 20 percent of Americans are burdened with overweight. We receive thousands of letters from doctors requesting exercise charts for their patients." He added, "If the mail is a true indicator, more women take the radio exercises than men; at least more women write than men. Of course, it may be that men ask the women to write for the charts. The men formerly wrote more than they do now. Sixty-five percent of the letters are from women."[42]

Physician Logan Clendening declared in one of his 1937 newspaper columns that more and more it was becoming the idea that simply cutting down food intake was all that was necessary to reduce while the use of exercise, massage, baths, or reducing drugs, did not contribute materially to the result. "Eat less and you will reduce: it is all very simple and mathematically logical," he exclaimed.[43]

Columnist Ida Kain regularly published reducing menus in her newspaper columns. Mostly, those diets were fairly severe, limiting the dieter to from 1,100 to 1,200 or so calories per day. A typical menu was as follows: Breakfast — half a glass of orange juice (50 calories); poached egg on toast (150); coffee, one teaspoon of cream, one rounded teaspoon of sugar (50); total calories of 250. Luncheon — one cup of vegetable soup (100); two rye wafers (40); pear and cottage cheese salad, fruit dressing (150); total calories of 290; snack — at 3:30 P.M. a glass of milk (80). Dinner — two ground round steak patties, broiled (200); half a cup of fresh lima beans (100); half a cup of beets (40); one pat of butter, .25 inches thick (50); tossed green salad, vinegar, seasoning, mineral oil (25); slices of pineapple (100); total calories of 515. Total calories for the day from this menu were 1,135. Readers were also advised to supplement the above menu with one Vitamin A, B, and D capsule.[44]

One of the few definitions of obesity in this period came from newspaper columnist Ida Kain in 1939 who stated that if a person weighed 20 percent more than specified by the actuarial tables for a person of that height and build then that person was obese.[45]

Logan Clendening returned later in 1939 to argue that in treating obesity, reliance was to be placed mainly on diet, "Extra exercise is not necessary; patients lose weight on a proper diet even if they remain in bed. Measurements of weight loss through exercise are somewhat misleading.

A football player may lose as much as 15 pounds during a game. But most of this is water loss. Only about a third of a pound is actual flesh. The water loss is regained within a few hours."[46]

Another of Ida Kain's low-calorie menus was published in her column on December 20, 1939, and read as follows: Breakfast — one glass of fresh or canned orange juice (110 calories); two thin slices of whole wheat toast (100); one pat of butter, .125 inches thick (50); total calories of 260. Luncheon — two scrambled eggs (215); two strips of crisp bacon (25); fresh or canned green vegetables (25); fruit (100); total calories of 365. Dinner — two pieces of pot roast (200); two whole carrots (50); broccoli and canned peas (50); grapefruit salad (50); three crackers (60); 1.125-inch cube of cheese (100); total calories of 510. Total calories for the day from the above menu were 1,135.

11

Style, Prevalence, and Statistics, 1920–1939

Reporter Mildred Holland wondered in a 1923 piece if her readers needed corsets. "A corset is a form of crutch. Only the woman whose flesh is so flabby that she must repress it in order to look trim should wear one," she said. One of the commonest misconceptions that fat women hold is the idea that they will look slimmer if they tighten their corsets so as to give them an inward curve at the small of the back. The effect is precisely opposite." Holland went on to say that the best way for a stout person to put on a corset was to lie flat on the back, "Any one large enough to need a corset at all needs to remember to pull the flesh up as much as possible underneath it. Most people push the flesh down." She went on to give a stretching exercise that was to be done by fat women before they put their corsets on.[1]

A brief review of a book in 1925 in the *Washington Post* remarked, "Now that the slender silhouette is the vogue of the moment in fashion circles, how to *Dress and Look Slender*, by Jane Warren Wells is a guide to the desired slimness no woman nearing the 'fair, fat and forty' stage can afford to overlook." According to the article there was no doubt that the requisite of slenderness had caused women lacking this quality "to resort to every known desire in the attempt, often with distressing experiences in the effort and with injurious effects upon the health." However, the reporter pointed out that relief was in sight for them because by proper dressing much of the effect of overweight could be dissipated by the application of certain "magic" principles of "optical illusions," worked out in a practical manner and presented so simply in the book by Wells that anyone could adopt them to her own requirements, "The author goes thoroughly into the subject. She tells just what gowns to wear, colors, shades, style of making up, materials, hats, shoes, corsets and type of lingerie."[2]

That same year, 1925, journalist Edward Folliard observed, "Obesity is the big bugaboo of the ladies who star in the movies. For that matter, I suppose, it is the bugaboo of almost all women. But the thought of becoming fat could never be as terrifying to a woman out of the movies as it must be to one who is in filmland." He added that to both, fleshiness meant the loss of a certain amount of charm and physical attractiveness. And that it was in the consequences of obesity that the great difference lay, "In the case of the movie star, one very probable consequence is the loss of her job and this means the loss of all that goes with it — fabulous wages, fame and public adulation. In short, obesity can mean ruin." It was said to be a given there was gossip in Hollywood when a screen star took on 10 pounds or so with the current rumor being centered on Nita Naldi. "Consequently, she has banished starchy foods from her table and has gone in for heavy exercise and rolling on the floor," explained Folliard. Other actors mentioned as being then threatened by obesity were Alice Terry, Leatice Joy, Barbara La Marr, and Linda Lee. The experiences of Lee were said to be a good example of the importance of keeping trim in the movies. Said Folliard, "The first time I saw her on the screen was in *Male and Female*. She was outrageously stout at the time, and as a consequence was cast in a more or less minor role. Three years later she had ridded herself of the superfluous flesh and was starring alongside Thomas Meighan."[3]

A dozen years later in 1937 Hollywood actresses were reported to be big on finding diets. Actor Glenda Farrell told a reporter she had tried five different recommended diets until she discovered that whenever she became a pound overweight the solution was to eat carrots. She could lose a pound by sticking to that diet for two days. Since she weighed herself daily, she never had more than one pound to take off. Anne Nagel, actor, explained that she never had to worry about the weight situation if she avoided eating when she was tired. Her explanation of that phenomenon was that because food could not be properly digested when a person was fatigued, it became fat. After a hard day's work at the studio she drank a quart of milk instead of eating solid food and her weight remained stationary. Marcia Ralston, actor, had the following ritual for maintaining her proper weight; each morning, before breakfast, she combined the juice of one medium-sized lemon with one tablespoon of honey and swallowed the mixture. It kept her weight down, she declared, but admitted she did not know why. However, it did not curb her appetite. As an added bonus, the mixture kept her complexion clear and glowing.[4]

In a 1934 article, reporter Virginia Lee Warren noted that overweight women "can create the illusion of slimness by choosing the right clothes; colors, materials, and lines play important parts." Warren declared that fashion "prophets" at frequent intervals in the previous six years had said that curves were back. But, with the exception of a few hectic weeks in the fall of 1933, when actor Mae West cast an "elephantine shadow" across the style landscape, every one of the prophecies was false. Designers had gone on creating silhouettes that were meant for "matchstick figures. Fashion artists have continued to depict the well-dressed woman as a tall, willowy creature. Most important of all, the slender, long-legged body is still considered the personification of youth, while plumpness is popularly supposed to represent maturity and stodginess." Also, remarked Warren, the woman with a few excess pounds here and there had a difficult time finding attractive clothes. Then the article went on to deal at length with the lines, colors, hats, materials, patterns, and so on (helped along by line drawings), best worn by overweight women, in order to make them look less fat.[5]

When the International Association of Clothing Designers issued its 1940 fashion forecast, in 1939, it declared that men's wearing apparel, such as suits, were designed to be more flattering to the overweight. Such new designs, it predicted, would benefit the corpulent man to a "greater degree than heretofore." This article was one of the very few that dealt with the subject of overweight men, fashion, and obesity.[6]

In the earlier periods covered by this book, from 1850 to 1919, there seemed to be no mentions of overweight children or teens in the literature. Thus, it appeared, that the problem did not exist. Only a little change was recorded in the period 1920 to 1939. For the first time, the press mentioned the topic of obese children, but those references were brief and few and far between. When Dr. Louis Bauman, director of the metabolism ward in Presbyterian Hospital in New York City, made his 1928 report about the treatment of obese patients at his institution he also warned mothers, in that report, to guard against overfeeding children in case overeating became a habit."[7]

Agnes Lyne authored a 1933 piece in the *Washington Post* called "Guiding your Child," which was perhaps the first article specifically about fat children. "To be a fat boy or a fat girl is frequently regarded simply as a joke, a difficulty which the child supposedly outgrows or which is 'in the family' and so can not be remedied. Depending upon the extent to which a child is overweight, this condition is to be regarded as a serious physical handicap, and as a social and psychological one," explained Lyne. Even though the fat child might develop a technique for handling ridicule it did not mean it did not bother him. Such children developed shyness, did not like to play in games where quickness and skill were important, and were shy about getting into a bathing suit. "At every turn, even though he is accepted by his age group, the overweight child is made to feel inferior, also tends to retire within himself. He does not try to compete with others of his age," added Lyne. "An overweight child should be taken to a doctor for diagnosis, and then should follow the course of treatment prescribed. Daily exercises and a dietary regime often are all that is necessary to bring his weight down to normal. Such exercising and dieting can only be carried on with cooperation from the parents, who have to accept the problem as an entirely serious one and help the child consistently to carry out the remedial regime."[8]

Columnist Ida Kain noted in 1939 "even in childhood overweight is a health handicap." Kain pointed out that child actor Shirley Temple had been on a diet and watched her weight as a matter of course. Around the same time Dr. Dafoe decided the Dionne quintuplets (born in Quebec in 1934 and the subject of huge media coverage) were overweight and he restricted the sugars and starches in their diet. In one month the five little girls lost from 0.5 pounds to 1.75 pounds each. "As a rule, overweight in childhood is apt to be dismissed as something that will be outgrown. If the habit of overeating is firmly established, however, it will grow up with the child," said Kain. "That is one reason why it is extremely important that children form the right food habits and that their parents help them." As far as Kain was concerned, any child who was more than 15 percent above the ideal weight for his age and height should be placed on a reducing diet.[9]

Hard, statistical data with respect to the number of overweight people there were in America remained elusive with most figures being vague, anecdotal estimates. Height and weight tables were readily available and heavily used in this period, and they provided a base of sorts from which to generate estimates of obesity rates that may have been marginally more revealing and helpful than estimates made prior to 1920, but only just. When fashion designer Paul Poiret's views on obesity were solicited in 1923 by a reporter, the latter observed, with respect to Poiret's view that clothing could not disguise a woman's fatness, "It is estimated that at least 40 per cent of the women in the United States will be dismayed and reduced to wailings and perhaps skin and bones by this statement. Nobody knows just now many women there are who could be classed as fat, but it is declared that almost half the women in the world accumulate some time during their lives more flesh than they ought to have."[10]

In an examination of the data from some 16,000 policyholders of the Metropolitan Life Insurance Company it was revealed that there were about 2,000 (12.5 percent) who were more than 20 percent overweight, that is, based on the average weight of people taking out life insurance.[11]

Doctor Leonard Williams advised people in 1926 to find out their "proper" weight by accepted standards (that is, the height and weight tables) and then to reduce themselves to a weight 20 pounds below it. He expressed dismay that those tables said a man at 25 should weigh 147 pounds and the same man at 50 should weight 162. Williams called the extra 15 pounds "lard superimposed" on the man of 25, "lard which has replaced muscle," and "it is useless and deleterious adipose tissue which has invaded and supplanted useful and necessary muscular tissue. It is not only an additional load; it is a degeneration." For Williams corpulence was not a comedy but a tragedy because it caused pain, disability, and inefficiency, and it shortened life, directly by clogging the wheels of being, indirectly by decreasing and weakening the powers of resistance. "The seemingly strong healthy man is the worst of all possible subjects for pneumonia, typhoid, or influenza, and no surgeon, however bold, will fear to declare that he dreads to operate upon a fat man," explained Williams. "Practically all the deaths under anesthetics have occurred among the corpulent."[12]

Weight and mortality statistics also became widely produced and widely disseminated in this period. Based on millions of observations from

Metropolitan Life data it was revealed in 1923 that among men 5'7" tall, 40 years old and weighing 184 pounds, the mortality rate was 30 percent above the norm; for men 5'7," 40, and 214 pounds, it was 80 percent higher than expected; for men 5'10," 40, 201 pounds, the mortality rate was 40 percent above the norm; for men 5'10," 40, 235 pounds, it was 100 percent higher. The proper weight for a 5'7" man of 40 was 153 pounds and for a 5'10" man of 40 it was 168 pounds. "This means that obesity is a health liability and one of major importance," said Dr. W. A. Evans. He used the age of 40 but the same results held true for every age period beyond 35. Up to 35 one could be a little overweight without being harmed thereby. By after the age of 35 it had an effect, "it is just that particular place in our journey through life that we begin to accumulate 'a fair round belly with good capon lined,' as friend Shakespeare has said." With respect to the standard weight tables, said Evans, "the standards of weights for given ages and heights represent averages. When we say a man 5 feet 7 inches, 40 years old, should weigh 153 pounds we mean that the average weight of a large number of people of that height and age was 153 pounds. The probability is that the average man is too fat, and therefore, that 153 pounds, while the average weight, is not the proper weight. The proper weight would be, say, 143 pounds."[13]

A lengthy 1931 article by insurance executive Louis Dublin had the scary title "Digging our Graves with our Teeth." He explained that for years the insurance fraternity had placed its chief reliance — with respect to the question as to how much a person should weigh — upon the so-called Medico-Actuarial Investigation of Build (the height/weight tables). The medical directors and actuaries of the leading insurance firms compiled a statistical report that covered the years 1885 to 1909. That report, said Dublin, "remains a classic on the relation between weight and mortality. It confirmed the general impression that overweight is a distinct handicap, the seriousness of which increases with the amount of excess and with age." The Standard Tables of Height and Weight, which accompanied Dublin's article (see Appendix A), were based directly on the Medico-Actuarial Investigation. That is, based on the height and weight data for people who successfully applied to life insurance firms for policies. Dublin believed the results from that study probably represented current conditions very well, despite the age of the data and "the recent reduction fad."[14]

After the data was collected, explained Dublin, the Metropolitan Life

Insurance Company then investigated the connection between weight and longevity. Studied were the records of nearly 200,000 white men from policies with the Union Central Life Insurance Company issued from 1887 to 1908, and who were then followed from the date their policies were issued up to 1921, or to an earlier date if their polices were terminated. Those 200,000 records were classified into nine groups, according to their height and weight at the time their insurance was written. Largest group was the so-called normal weight group, people that varied less than five percent, plus or minus, from the average as given in the Standard Tables. Plus there were five groups of overweight people and three groups of underweight policyholders. For analysis, explained Dublin, only three classes of overweight were used; five to fifteen percent above, 15 to 25 percent, and over 25 percent above. Only two classes of underweight were used; five to 15 percent low, 15 to 34 percent under. The subsequent mortality of each of those six groups was then followed. With the death rate of the normal weight group given the arbitrary value of 100 then the mortality rate for the underweight class as a whole was also 100, but for the overweights as a whole it was 132. For the two underweight groups the rates were 99 (five to 15 percent group) and 108; for the three overweight groups the numbers were, respectively from least to most obese, 122, 144, and 174. Age was also a factor, with the groups subdivided into under 45 and over 45. Among younger men, those of average weight showed the lowest death rates with young underweights at 108 and young overweights at 114. Young men, extremely underweight showed a mortality rate of 116; mortality of the young and slightly overweight was 110. Above the age of 45 underweights as a whole had a mortality rate as a whole of 97, slightly underweights stood at 96. As a whole the old overweights had a mortality rate of 139; for the three overweight groups. Lowest to highest respectively, the numbers were 127, 156, 186. Dublin pointed out that all of those overweight men in the study were the "best" of the obese as they had all successfully qualified for life insurance. That is, if the mortality rate for all obese men had been included (adding in those rejected for insurance) then the mortality rate would have been higher. With respect to the height/weight tables, Dublin said, "In general, then, it is wise for people to keep within the figures of the Standard Tables, and after they are thirty-five it would be better if they could lop off a few pounds from the normal." He also noted that in a study of over 200,000 records of examination made by the Life Extension Institute among apparently well people it was found that almost 13 percent were at least 20 percent overweight. "At present too many of us are digging our graves with our teeth. We can add years to our lives and happiness to our days if we take to heart the lessons on the relation between weight and longevity which these figures of the statistician have disclosed," Dublin concluded.[15]

A new study of the relationship of weight to physical defects was published in 1933 by the U.S. Public Health Service. By the time that middle age was reached, it was declared to be a definite advantage to be under the average weight for height, said the report. It also revealed "a great excess of mortality among overweight persons, whatever the age, and also an excess among young adult underweight persons." Conclusions were drawn from records of more than 3,000 men over the period 1909 to 1928, showing the ratio of actual deaths to expected mortality, according to different weight groups. The expected death rates for the normal weight groups were all set arbitrarily at 100. Mortality rates for those 25 or more pounds underweight were as follows: 20 to 29 years, 118; 30 to 39, 105; 40 to 49, 83; 50 plus, 77. For men 10 to 20 pounds underweight, 101, 94, 76, 85; for those 10 to 20 pounds overweight, 99, 88, 94, 90; for those 25 to 45 pounds overweight, 113, 123, 125, 119; and for those people 50 and more pounds overweight, 163, 143, 144, 130. Overweight people had the worst of it in an analysis of the death rate from 15 different causes; only tuberculosis showed any marked excess mortality among underweight people. On the other hand, a large number of causes of death primarily degenerative in nature, showed an excess among overweight people. Organic heart disease deaths among those over 45 were 253 per 100,000 for men 50 pounds or more overweight; 213 for normal weight; 161 for those 25 pounds and more underweight. Other causes of death with higher frequency among the obese men included appendicitis, cirrhosis of the liver, and diabetes. Another was death from brain hemorrhage and apoplexy wherein among men over 45 years of age the death rate was 156 deaths per 100,000 for the overweights, 118 for the normal weight group; and 67 for the underweight group.[16]

According to an analysis of health statistics of 336,000 people made in 1934 by Louis Dublin, 20 percent of all Americans were overweight or underweight. The study revealed that if a person was under 30 years of age it was a real health advantage to weigh at least 10 percent more than average. For those over 35 years of age, being moderately underweight (about 10 percent below average) indicated a longer life than average. Women aged 25 who were 20 percent below average weight had a death rate 11 percent greater than average while women over 35 who were 10 percent overweight had a death rate 22 percent above average. If they weighed 25 percent above the average the mortality rate jumped to 74 percent above normal, shortening life by 6.5 years.[17]

A few years later, in 1937, columnist Ida Kain mentioned the work of Louis Dublin on longevity and weight, stating, "The weight tendency of the average woman is in direct contradiction to the laws of health and longevity. Instead of maintaining normal weight or, as recommended, a weight that is slightly under the accepted average after the age of 30, she continues to take on excess pounds." Kain said that according to Dublin's figures, the average weight gain was three pounds for women between the ages of 25 and 35; seven pounds between 30 and 40, and six pounds between 40 and 50. Thus, if a woman experienced an average weight gain she would be 16 pounds over the weight of her 25-year-old self when she reached the age of 50. With regard to the height/weight tables Kain said, "It is difficult to tell what your normal weight should be. Even the weight charts allow for a gradual increase as you grow older. Do not overlook the fact, however, that these charts are based on average weights and not on normal weight for the individual." Dublin criticized the tables because they did not take into account variation in body structure (that is, small, medium, and large bone structure) and argued that structure as well as height should be the basis for computing normal weight. Dublin's rule for determining "normal" weight was as follows: a small-boned individual should allow 100 pounds for five feet of height; 105 pounds for a medium-size frame; and 110 pounds if the frame was large, for the first five feet of height. Then, for all cases, add 5.5 pounds for each inch of height exceeding five feet.[18]

Ida Kain declared, in 1939, that there were about seven women who weighed too much for every overweight man. Reportedly that estimate came from a number of large obesity clinics and was confirmed by the registration at a famous New York hospital that gave special attention to weight reduction. The greater frequency of obesity among women was said to be explained by their more sedentary lives.[19]

Conclusion

Over the period 1850 to 1939 obesity in American moved from being a virtually non-existent issue to one that was much discussed in the media, with columnists both medical and lay pondering the topic in the daily newspapers and the magazines. By the 1930s in America weight reduction was undertaken by many people in society, formally and informally, but mostly by women. Perhaps 20 percent of the population suffered from fatness in the 1920s and 1930s in the U.S.A., although estimates were vague and unclear and operational definitions were largely absent. Quackery was a part of the obesity industry, throughout this entire period, and remained so into the 21st century. People spent months and years getting to be obese but mostly did not want to spend an equal amount of time and effort in getting their weight back to normal. And so the quick and effortless fix offered by most quack remedies ensured quackery a steady trade despite its mostly being obvious nonsense. Various bizarre, erroneous ideas as to the cause of obesity took hold in the early years covered in this book. Some of them — such as zero-calorie tap water being fattening — have long since vanished from current popular articles on being overweight. However, some have remained — such as the idea that certain foods were fattening (with no consideration given to caloric value). The potato was one example, although there were others.

During the 1850 to 1879 period there were very few mentions of obesity in the media. While a media did exist it was not nearly as large and flourishing as it would be a few decades later. The relatively higher cost of newspapers and magazines and the higher illiteracy rates in this period made the media less accessible. As well, obesity was a problem initially for the upper class (it later spread downward) and while the problems of the upper class have often been presented in the media as the problems of society as a whole, the upper class of the 1850s and 1860s, say, was still relatively weak and did not then draw the fawning attention of the press that the upper class would in, say, the 1890s. Mostly though, the vast majority of Americans in the period 1850 to 1879 led hard, physical lives. Obesity was only rarely mentioned because it likely hardly existed. Still, some stereotypes associated with fatness existed even then. Some adjectives associated with obesity included jolly, laughing, honest, lazy, and not too bright. Emphasized was that the obese were disproportionately not criminal. If the idea of the Rubenesque figure being beautiful and sexually attractive had ever had any currency in America, it had left the nation before 1850. Obesity, as well, was said to affect the sexes differently with the condition hurting women's attractiveness and hurting the ability of men to perform at work. A recognition that overweight was bad for the health in general existed, but it was rudimentary and did not usually mention the diseases that would later become linked to the condition — and would remain so into the 21st century. It was generally agreed that a large amount of fat on a person diminished bodily and mental activity.

During the period 1850 to 1879 there was the emergence of the so-called dime museums, which featured various human oddities — the "freaks" in the "freak shows" — put on public display. One of the staples in all such shows was the fat woman and/or the fat man. The listed weights for such behemoths were usually wildly exaggerated. Additionally, newspapers regularly ran brief articles about the grossly fat that were not on display for profit, in various "human interest" situations. No real science of obesity could be said to exist in this period. It was all quackery with some of that coming from quacks and some of it coming from the respectable medical and scientific communities. Causes advanced to explain obesity included heredity, too much sleep, a constant breathing of damp air, and too much drinking of fluids (zero-calorie water and relatively high-calorie beer were considered to be the same, both were fluids and had the same effect on the body). The idea that a major cause of obesity lay in consuming too much food was not absent, but it was a minority view. With respect to reducing, the drastic method of surgery to remove fat was mentioned but, presumably, not much used. One diet advanced, with variations, by different medical men had the patient living mainly on meat and drinking only a little liquid (and none of that being water). Spa waters, soap pills, and eating very few vegetables were other recommendations. Clubs for fat men sprang up all over America in this period. Mostly such clubs were social in nature and afforded their members the opportunity on one or more occasions each year to gather and participate in eating a gargantuan meal. No accounts surfaced as to the prevalence of obesity in America then but a few anecdotal articles pointed out that many fat women were to be found in the resort areas where the elite took their vacations. Reinforced was the idea that whatever obesity there was in America in 1850 to 1879 was to be found mainly in the upper class. There was no such thing, apparently, as a fat child.

Over the years 1880 to 1919 many more articles devoted to obesity appeared in the media. For the first time the topic began to appear in columns. With respect to the science of obesity the period was one of transition, with all quackery at the beginning but by the end of World War I the quackery came mostly from the quacks. Respectable science and medicine offered more coherent, logical, and accurate thoughts on the matter. Several articles appeared that argued fat people could be geniuses too, but since each such article tended to cite the same few people as examples, those articles, taken as a group, were less than convincing. Stressed again was that overweight people rarely became criminals; fat people were still seen as lazy. Actresses were felt to be finished on the stage if they ever got to be obese, illustrating perhaps, a public dislike of obesity. Public figures such as German kaiser Wilhelm and U.S. presidents William Taft and Grover Cleveland all tried to reduce and their efforts at weight control were closely followed by the media. Fat people were not popular in real life, in the literary world, or on the theatrical stage. Obese people had less blood, they breathed differently; they were cautious and conservative; they ate a lot and slept a lot; the idea of a fat lover was a joke. On the other hand, fat people were said to endure most illnesses better than did the normal and thin people. Jolliness and stoutness were generally found together; all stout people were not jolly, but nearly all jolly people were stout.

Clubs for fat men continued to be popular in the years 1880 to 1919. Displays of fat people, and other freaks, in dime museums lessened greatly in popularity as vaudeville overwhelmed the museums. Many athletic events were held for fat men, usually at the annual summer event —

picnic or field day — of one large organization or another, such as the 100-yard race for fat men. Especially prevalent were such races at the yearly police athletic games held by police departments all over America. A few mentions surfaced that discussed the difficulties fat men had in getting work — employers worried the fat man was lazy, soft, and so on. By the end of this period, 1916, the New York Civil Service Commission, as part of a crackdown on widespread municipal corruption, nepotism, and so on, instituted uniform civil service rules for job applicants. One bar, in some areas, was obesity. For the first time, fatness was an official and formal bar to employment.

Nonsense abounded in the years 1880 to 1919, with regard to the cause of obesity, at least in the early years of the period. Ordinary tap water continued to be cited as fattening by medical men; fatness was inherited, exposure to the sun prevented obesity. More and more the idea of "fat and healthy" fell into disfavor. Standing incorrectly caused fatness. Alcohol caused obesity, as did nervous disorders. Too much automobile riding caused fatness, but not for the expected reason that it curtailed walking but because the angle of the seats caused muscles to relax and the exhilaration that rapid movement produced and the increase in appetite from the open air moved a person toward obesity. Many women's columnists (who wrote on beauty hints, and so on) often discussed obesity. And it was from that area that many bizarre notions sprang, including the idea that the cause of fatness in the 25 to 30-year-old woman different from the cause of fatness in women around the age of 40. Celebrities sometimes weighed in on the subject. Actor superstar Lillian Russell argued heredity was the cause, as did many others. Many theories evolved that centered on food as cause, such as the potato being bad. No less an authority than the U.S. government, through its Agriculture Department, had a cure for obesity, in 1907. That involved eating little, sleeping little, and drinking less fluid. No water was to be consumed within one hour, plus/minus, of mealtime, preferably two hours. Patients were told to give up food such as peas, beets, cauliflower, cabbage, parsnips, bananas, and so on, and to eat only the three or four vegetables that thinned the blood. And, from other quarters, came the posture cure, the stooping cure, the somersault cure, the standing cure, and the surgery cure was still around. Only a few mentions were made of exercise as a possible remedy for obesity. Exercise could be a worry for women because it hardened them, made them muscular and that was decidedly not feminine. Platinum injections enjoyed the status of being a fad, for a very brief time while electrical stimulation of the muscles to reduce weight had a somewhat longer fad status. A selling point for electrical stimulation was that it offered something for nothing, that is, weight reduction with no effort or sacrifice on the part of the patient.

Advice for obesity treatment in the years 1880 to 1919 usually centered on diet alone, although a few accounts added some words that exercise could help as an addition to diet. Only a small handful of articles dealt with exercise alone as a treatment for obesity. Specific diets and menus were regularly published in the media for the guidance of the general public but the specific amounts of food to be consumed were usually lacking. Occasionally a menu specified six ounces of lean beef but more usually it just said to eat lean mutton, or cucumbers, and so on. Fruits were usually praised as good foods to eat for those trying to reduce but, for unstated reasons, the banana joined the potato as one of the items to make most of the blacklists. Bread was the other food on the list of the top three items to be avoided. Another minor craze was to eat just one item at each meal, only spinach, or only beef, and so on. The idea of best foods, bad foods, fattening foods, and so forth, remained strong in this period (again, with caloric value ignored). Increasingly, around 1900 and thereafter, articles on obesity and reducing were directed solely at women, over and above those directed at the general population; there were no articles on obesity aimed at men only. Only at the end of this period were there a few articles on caloric value of food items. Science had improved and knowing the caloric value of food items meant that diet advice could be more precise and more accurate. Also taking hold late in this period more and more was the idea that obesity resulted from eating too much and exercising too little, that is, it was a matter of calories in and calories out. However, it was still a minority position, but growing in acceptance.

Most accounts of the prevalence of fat people in the years 1880 to 1919 were also vague and anecdotal. A few more reports from resorts for the elite confirmed the idea that fatness was fairly common among the upper class. Late in this period the height/weight tables took hold and soon became a pervasive part of American society. Articles about fashion and obesity turned up in this period and soon became commonplace. Some talked about the lack of stylish clothes for fat women and some talked about what types of clothing those fat women should wear in order to appear slimmer. Anecdotally, the prevalence of fat people was said to have increased by the late 1880s over, say 1850. Life insurance data from those who had taken out policies began to receive widespread use — for the height/weight tables, and for mortality rates. Hard evidence then existed to show that obesity was a killer. Also, the idea became ingrained in society that there were many more fat women in America than fat men. There was no such thing, apparently, as a fat child.

During the final years covered by this book, 1920 to 1939, the image that fat people were lazy, could not be lovers, were honest, and had less participation in the crime rates continued to appear. Freaks faded away almost entirely as did the fat men's clubs and the fat men's races. In employment there was more pressure on police officers not to be fat. Attributions of obesity to silly and strange causes from respectable members of the medical and scientific communities were almost gone. Calories in and calories out as the cause had achieved almost complete acceptance. This period marked the first time that articles on obesity could be found that dealt exclusively with the diseases and health effects from being fat — with high blood pressure, diabetes, and heart disease leading the way. Fatness was declared to be a dangerous and risky state.

Obesity in this period was seen as a big enough topic that it became a public health issue with high profile and well-publicized reduction efforts launched by the health departments in the cities of Chicago and New York. Metropolitan Life Insurance Company became perhaps the first company to offer an in-house weight reduction program for its employees. Exercising got somewhat more emphasis as a way to reduce weight but it still took a back seat to diet. Reducing became a big fad as hospitals, clinics, and adult education officials set up weight reduction programs. Even more books and articles on fashion and obesity made their appearance. More detailed use was made of height/weight tables and mortality rates. There were still no reliable or useable figures on the prevalence of fat people in America. For the first time a very few specific articles were printed that mentioned fat children.

Appendix: Average Weights
of Men and Women (1931)

Average Weights of Men

Height (with shoes on)	Weight in Pounds According to Age (as ordinarily dressed)								
	15–19	*20–24*	*25–29*	*30–34*	*35–39*	*40–44*	*45–49*	*50–54*	*55–59*
5'0"	113	119	124	127	129	132	134	135	136
5'1"	115	121	126	129	131	134	136	137	138
5'2"	118	124	128	131	133	136	138	139	140
5'3"	121	127	131	134	136	139	141	142	143
5'4"	124	131	134	137	140	142	144	145	146
5'5"	128	135	138	141	144	146	148	149	150
5'6"	132	139	142	145	148	150	152	153	154
5'7"	136	142	146	149	152	154	156	157	158
5'8"	140	146	150	154	157	159	161	162	163
5'9"	144	150	154	158	162	164	166	167	168
5'10"	148	154	158	163	167	169	171	172	173
5'11"	153	158	163	168	172	175	177	178	179
6'0"	158	163	169	174	178	181	183	184	185
6'1"	163	168	175	180	184	187	190	191	192
6'2"	168	173	181	186	191	194	197	198	199

Appendix

AVERAGE WEIGHTS OF WOMEN

Height (with shoes on)	Weight in Pounds According to Age (as ordinarily dressed)								
	15–19	20–24	25–29	30–34	35–39	40–44	45–49	50–54	55–59
4'11"	110	113	116	119	122	126	129	131	132
5'0"	112	115	118	121	124	128	131	133	134
5'1"	114	117	120	123	126	130	133	135	137
5'2"	117	120	122	125	129	133	136	138	140
5'3"	120	123	125	128	132	136	139	141	143
5'4"	123	126	129	132	136	139	142	144	146
5'5"	126	129	132	136	140	143	146	148	150
5'6"	130	133	136	140	144	147	151	152	153
5'7"	134	137	140	144	148	151	155	157	158
5'8"	138	141	144	148	152	155	159	162	163
5'9"	141	145	148	152	156	159	163	166	167
5'10"	145	149	152	155	159	162	166	170	173
5'11"	150	153	155	158	162	166	170	174	177
6'0"	155	157	169	162	165	169	173	177	182

Source: Louis I. Dublin, "Digging our graves with our teeth." The Forum and Century 85 (May 1931): 314–5.

Chapter Notes

Chapter 1

1. "Rather fat." *Brooklyn Eagle*, January 7, 1850, p. 2.
2. "The art of unfattening." *Brooklyn Eagle*, June 20, 1857, p. 1.
3. *Ibid.*
4. *Ibid.*
5. "Corpulency." *Brooklyn Eagle*, April 17, 1863, p. 1.
6. "Fat and felony." *Brooklyn Eagle*, July 5, 1865, p. 1.
7. Corry O'Lanus. "Corry O'Lanus' epistle." *Brooklyn Eagle*, November 27, 1869, p. 2.
8. "Auxiliary fat men." *New York Times*, February 24, 1877, p. 4.
9. "Death from obesity." *Hartford Courant*, September 15, 1853, p. 2.
10. "Local matters." *The Union Vedette* (Utah), February 4, 1865, p. 3.
11. "The art of unfattening." *Brooklyn Eagle*, June 20, 1857, p. 1.
12. *Ibid.*
13. *Ibid.*
14. *Ibid.*
15. "Corpulency." *Brooklyn Eagle*, April 17, 1863, p. 1.
16. "Fat people." *Liberty Weekly Tribune* (Missouri), October 6, 1871, p. 1.
17. "Risk of great eaters." *The Hillsdale Standard* (Michigan), August 7, 1866.
18. "Sleep and grow fat." *Hornellsville Tribune* (Steuben County, N. Y.), March 4, 1870, p. 1.
19. "Fat and fashionable." *Rocky Mountain News* (Denver), September 18, 1875, p. 3.
20. "A British disease." *Washington Post*, April 17, 1879, p. 3.
21. "Are fat people healthy." *Boulder News and Courier* (Colorado), April 25, 1879, p. 1.
22. "The Fat Men's Association." *New York Times*, November 24, 1869, p. 5.
23. "Fat men's ball." *New York Times*, December 21, 1869, p. 8.
24. "The jolly fat men of Brooklyn." *New York Times*, December 19, 1869, p. 8.
25. "The German fat men's target excursion." *New York Times*, June 22, 1870, p. 5.
26. "Stout parties' picnic." *New York Times*, August 20, 1870, p. 2.

27. "Fat men in Put-in-Bay." *Ohio Democrat* (New Philadelphia), August 23, 1872; "The fat men's convention." *Richmond Gazette* (Ohio), September 11, 1873.

28. "The clam gourmands." *New York Times*, August 28, 1874, p. 5.

29. "Fat men on a frolic." *New York Times*, August 24, 1877, p. 8.

30. "Fat men eating clams." *New York Times*, September 5, 1879, p. 5.

Chapter 2

1. "A comfort to fat people." *Chester Daily Times* (Pennsylvania), June 21, 1880.

2. "Human obesity." *The Indiana Democrat* (Indiana, Pennsylvania), August 2, 1883, p. 1.

3. "A lower berth." *The Oxford Mirror* (Oxford Junction, Iowa), October 4, 1883.

4. "The evolution of the corset." *New York Times*, May 11, 1884, p. 11.

5. "The terrors of obesity." *Brooklyn Eagle*, November 1, 1885, p. 6.

6. "Fat men East and West." *San Juan Prospector* (Del Norte, Colorado), January 23, 1886, p. 4.

7. "Obesity vs. independence." *Los Angeles Times,* April 8, 1891, p. 7.

8. "Undue corpulency." *Colorado Transcript* (Golden, Jefferson County), August 2, 1893, p. 7.

9. "Fat footpads." *Los Angeles Times*, January 29, 1905, sec 2, p. 8.

10. "More fat rogues than lean." *Los Angeles Times*, December 23, 1906, sec 7, p. 4.

11. "Most rulers have tendency to fat." *Washington Post*, January 24, 1909, p. E4.

12. Alma Whitaker. "Are fat men dangerous?" *Los Angeles Times*, December 23, 1913, sec 2, p. 4.

13. Blanche Beacon. "Little beauty chats." *Los Angeles Times*, April 14, 1914, sec 2, p. 5.

14. "Fat men unpopular now." *Akron Weekly Pioneer Press* (Colorado), April 17, 1914, p. 6.

15. "What car pleases fat men and lean men?" *Los Angeles Times*, September 24, 1916, sec 6, p. 9.

16. "The fat and the lean." *Brooklyn Eagle*, April 1, 1887, p. 2.

17. "Indebted to our fat men." *San Antonio Daily Light*, November 2, 1888.

18. "Intellect and obesity." *Washington Post*, April 27, 1890. p. 19.

19. "The disadvantages of obesity." *Hartford Courant*, May 16, 1891, p. 4.

20. No title. *Boulder Daily Camera* (Colorado), June 17, 1893, p. 2.

21. "Personal gossip." *Greeley Tribune* (Colorado), October 26, 1893, p. 9.

22. "Some consolation." *Colorado Transcript* (Golden, Jefferson County), December 6, 1893, p. 3.

23. "Fat women." *Grand Valley Times* (Utah), December 25, 1896.

24. "Good word for fat men." *Washington Post*, October 8, 1904, p. 9.

25. "Corpulency and sanity." *The Park Record* (Utah), January 13, 1906.

26. "Grow prosperous: fatten your wife." *Oakland Tribune*, January 4, 1907, p. 14.

27. "Smile of fat men sadder than tears." *Oakland Tribune*, May 3, 1908, p. 18.

28. "Consolation for the fat." *Washington Post*, May 24, 1908, p. SM3.

29. "Corpulence and genius." *Washington Post*, March 25, 1914, p. 6.

30. "Fat men of genius." *Washington Post*, February 13, 1916, p. S4.
31. "Laughing makes you fat." *Washington Post*, October 22, 1916, p. MT8.

Chapter 3

1. "Fat women." *New York Times*, October 6, 1881, p. 4.
2. "Human obesity." *New York Times*, August 18, 1883, p. 3.
3. "How fat people are made." *Washington Post*, December 26, 1883, p. 2.
4. "A talk about freaks." *Brooklyn Eagle*, September 24, 1887, p. 6.
5. "She weighs 650 pounds." *Salt Lake Tribune*, March 3, 1889, p. 5.
6. "Giants and fat men." *New York Times*, March 19, 1905, p. 8.
7. "Says fat women pay." *Los Angeles Times*, July 23, 1911, sec 5, p. 20.
8. "Fast fat men." *New York Times*, May 25, 1884, p. 3.
9. "Holmes' Star Theater." *Brooklyn Eagle*, August 24, 1890, p. 9.
10. "Law for fat men." *New York Times*, January 30, 1898, p. 21.
11. "To tax fat people." *Breckenridge Bulletin* (Colorado), July 25, 1903, p. 5.
12. "Chicago men arrange to have obesity club." *Oakland Tribune*, April 15, 1907, p. 3.
13. "The big man's year." *Washington Post*, June 17, 1908, p. 17.
14. "Slavery in sweatshops of Paris is revolting." *Oakland Tribune*, April 12, 1908, p. 26.
15. "Fat people blocked traffic on stairs." *Ogden Standard Examiner* (Utah), July 29, 1908.
16. "Fat people in protest." *The Wasatch Wave* (Utah), August 21, 1908, p. 4.
17. "Portly bridal couple." *Los Angeles Times*, December 10, 1911, p. 4.
18. "Appeal to Teutons at Irish bazaar." *New York Times*, October 15, 1916, p. 9.
19. "Too much of Flushing." *New York Times*, October 9, 1885, p. 3.
20. "San Diego County." *Los Angeles Times*, November 30, 1897, p. 13.
21. "No fat men for football." *New York Times*, March 20, 1905, p. 9.
22. "Catholic picnic." *Los Angeles Times*, August 26, 1897, p. 6.
23. "Angelino tots win ribbons." *Los Angeles Times*, August 5, 1906, p. 18.
24. "Sheridan was third in policemen's games." *New York Times*, August 8, 1906, p. 4.
25. "French are gay on Bastille day." *Los Angeles Times*, July 15, 1911, sec 2, p. 3.
26. "Bees buzz and all are happy." *Los Angeles Times*, July 28, 1911, p. 14.
27. "There was fun for everyone." *Los Angeles Times*, August 20, 1911, p. 8.
28. "Fat men are main eventers." *Los Angeles Times*, August 16, 1913, sec 4, p. 2.
29. "The glory of adipose." *New York Times*, August 28, 1884, p. 5.
30. "Outing of the Fat Men's Club." *Washington Post*, June 20, 1893, p. 2.
31. "Jolly fat men parade." *Washington Post*, September 1, 1893, p. 2.
32. "Fun of the fat men." *Washington Post*, July 9, 1894, p. 6.
33. "Our quota of club freaks." *Los Angeles Times*, August 1, 1897, p. 17.
34. "A policeman's happy lot." *New York Times*, June 17, 1882, p. 2.
35. "Traffic officers' field day games." *New York Times*, August 2, 1915, p. 7.
36. "Policemen in trouble." *Washington Post*, July 12, 1894, p. 6.
37. "Were members of the club." *Washington Post*, July 15, 1894, p. 2.
38. "Ten coppers dropped." *Washington Post*, August 17, 1894, p. 8.
39. "His baton restored." *Washington Post*, December 5, 1897, p. 3.

40. "No old, short, fat men need apply." *Fort Collins Weekly Courier* (Colorado), April 11, 1906, p. 9.

41. Willard W. Garrison. "Chicago has 5,000 policemen-athletes." *Kiowa County Press* (Eads, Colorado), October 30, 1908, p. 6.

42. "Bingham sued for $100,000." *Washington Post*, June 4, 1910, p. 4.

43. "Gen. Shafter on fat men." *Los Angeles Times*, December 9, 1906, sec 7, p. 5.

44. "France may call fat men." *New York Times*, June 21, 1915, p. 2.

45. "Fat men and jobs." *Los Angeles Times*, October 27, 1907, sec 2, p. 4.

46. "Thin fire brigade." *New York Times*, November 22, 1908, p. C4.

47. "Call stage heavyweights." *New York Times*, March 1, 1909, p. 9.

48. "Obesity a bar to office." *New York Times*, February 9, 1916, p. 12.

49. "No jobs for fat men there." *Lincoln Daily News* (Nebraska), July 1, 1916, p. 4.

Chapter 4

1. "Human obesity." *The Indiana Democrat* (Indiana, Pennsylvania), August 2, 1883, p. 1.

2. "Fat people and fluids." *Brooklyn Eagle*, October 11, 1886, p. 2.

3. "Hints about health." *Hartford Courant*, September 6, 1888, p. 2.

4. "Scientific miscellany." *Montezuma Millrun* (Summit County, Colorado), February 25, 1888, p. 3.

5. "How not to get too fat." *Washington Post*, March 5, 1888, p. 4.

6. "The Victorian obesity." *Leadville Daily and Evening Chronicle* (Colorado), June 5, 1888, p. 1.

7. "Too solid flesh." *The Rolla New Era* (Missouri), December 26, 1896, p. 4.

8. W. R. C. Latson. "Methods of reducing obesity." *Los Angeles Times*, September 1, 1903, p. A3.

9. "Drink habit." *The Lowell Sun* (Massachusetts), September 23, 1903, p. 5.

10. "Why drinkers are fat." *Littleton Independent* (Colorado), December 31, 1915, p. 6.

11. "How to get thin." *New York Times*, May 14, 1907, p. 10.

12. "Motoring spoils figure." *Washington Post*, January 9, 1910, p. A13.

13. Lina Cavalieri. "My secrets of beauty." *Washington Post*, October 8, 1911, p. E9.

14. Lillian Russell. "How to keep from getting fat." *Oakland Tribune*, October 9, 1913.

15. R. P. Daniels. "Obesity — its cause and cure." *Box Elder News* (Utah), February 2, 1914, p. 6.

16. "The potato habit." *Washington Post*, August 23, 1914, p. M3.

17. "Number of fat women is appalling." *Washington Post*, April 25, 1915, p. E14.

18. "Overfeeding causes obesity." *Haswell Herald* (Colorado), March 8, 1917, p. 2.

19. "The three planes of living." *Literary Digest* 54 (April 7, 1917): 977–978.

20. "How to cure obesity." *Washington Post*, November 15, 1885, p. 7.

21. "Fat folks turn somersaults." *Aspen Tribune* (Colorado), November 22, 1896, p. 2.

22. "Testing a new obesity cure." *New York Times*, September 25, 1898, p. 22.

23. "Lord Rodney, wife beater." *Los Angeles Times*, March 23, 1902, p. A15.

24. "A godsend to all humanity." *Los Angeles Times*, January 29, 1899, p. B5.

25. "Hope for the fat folks." *Hartford Courant*, August 30, 1899, p. 8.

26. "An obesity cure from Europe." *Washington Post*, April 3, 1900, p. 3.

27. "To reduce the abdomen." *Daily Journal* (Telluride, Colorado), August 28, 1901, p. 4.

28. Christine Terhune Herrick. "The Times' answers by experts." *Los Angeles Times*, July 3, 1902, p. A5.

29. "Fasting for corpulent people." *Emery County Progress* (Utah), May 10, 1902.

30. "Don't be fat." *Washington Post*, March 24, 1904, p. 8.

31. "Are too many fat and lean." *Los Angeles Times*, April 9, 1907, p. 3.

32. "She has corset cure." *Washington Post*, February 27, 1908, p. 2.

33. "Fat woman pared down by surgeons." *Oakland Tribune*, June 13, 1908.

34. "Hints for fat persons." *New York Times*, May 14, 1909, p. 11.

35. "The housemothers' exchange." *Los Angeles Times*, June 20, 1909, sec 6, p. 2.

36. "Anti-fat and society women." *Durango Wage Earner* (Colorado), October 26, 1911, p. 3.

37. Ada Lee. "Loses fat — wins fortune." *Washington Post*, April 16, 1912, p. 12.

38. *Ibid.*

39. *Ibid.*

40. "Indict beauty doctors." *New York Times*, June 7, 1912, p. 8.

41. "Stout women turned down." *Los Angeles Times*, June 26, 1913, p. 6.

42. No title. *Daily Journal* (Telluride, Colorado), June 28, 1913, p. 1.

43. "Tapeworm pills for fat people merely a wild yarn, say experts." *Washington Post*, December 6, 1912, p. 5.

44. "Fake anti-fat cure worries government." *Washington County News* (Utah), November 26, 1914.

45. Lina Cavalieri. "Mme. Cavalieri tells of a new obesity treatment." *Washington Post*, January 19, 1913, p. MT7.

46. "Reduction of obesity." *Los Angeles Times*, August 22, 1913, sec 2, p. 1.

47. "Has new rule for meals." *Washington Post*, April 27, 1914, p. 7.

48. "Fat people shouldn't wear clothes." *Washington Post*, October 5, 1913, p. MT8.

49. "Platinum cure for obesity." *New York Times*, January 18, 1914, p. C2.

50. "Baroness Suttner, peace leader, dies." *New York Times*, June 22, 1914, p. 4.

51. "To fat people." *Manti Messenger* (Utah), August 7, 1914, p. 8.

Chapter 5

1. "What determination will do." *Washington Post*, September 29, 1882, p. 2.

2. "Fat and lean people." *The Galveston Daily News*, December 26, 1882.

3. "The brigand treatment." *New York Times*, January 6, 1884, p. 6.

4. "Fat as a cure for obesity." *New York Times*, May 2, 1884, p. 2.

5. "The proper weight of man." *The Penn Yan Express* (Penn Yan, New York), November 5, 1884.

6. "Humorous." *Fort Collins Courier* (Colorado), May 28, 1885, p. 1.

7. "Reduction of fat." *The Oxford Mirror* (Oxford Junction, Iowa), November 26, 1886.

8. *Ibid.*

9. John Wilson Gibbs. "Ridding Cleveland of fat." *Salt Lake Tribune*, July 9, 1893, p. 15.

10. *Ibid.*

11. *Ibid.*

12. *Ibid.*

13. "To reduce one's weight." *Washington Post*, June 2, 1901, p. 23.

14. "An awful tale." *Washington Post*, May 31, 1885, p. 4.

15. "Useful hints to fleshy people." *Liberty Weekly Tribune* (Missouri), June 26, 1885, p. 1.

16. "Value of fruit." *The Rolla New Era* (Missouri), April 23, 1887, p. 4.

17. "Fat is the question." *The Galveston Daily News*, April 30, 1889, p. 6.

18. *Ibid.*

19. "Obesity and la grippe." *New York Times*, January 22, 1890, p. 3.

20. "How to cure obesity." *Castle Rock Journal* (Colorado), December 30, 1891, p. 3.

21. "Of interest to fat people." *New York Times*, September 24, 1893, p. 10.

22. "Another way to reduce flesh." *New York Times*, October 8, 1893, p. 18.

23. "Undue corpulency." *Colorado Transcript* (Golden, Jefferson County), August 2, 1893, p. 7.

24. "Quick lunches make fat men." *Los Angeles Times*, April 25, 1896, p. 14.

25. "A bad county." *Rifle Reveille* (Rifle, Colorado), August 7, 1896, p. 3.

26. "Fat women." *Grand Valley Times* (Utah), December 25, 1896.

27. "Kelp is eaten by Californians as a salad." *Daily Journal* (Telluride, Colorado), March 21, 1898, p. 3.

28. "How stout women may grow thin." *Washington Post*, July 10, 1898, p. 17.

29. "Fat women and thin ones." *Colorado Transcript* (Golden, Jefferson County), August 10, 1898, p. 3.

30. "Fruit to reduce flesh." *Washington Post*, December 18, 1898, p. 30.

31. "The true story of obesity." *Salt Lake Tribune* (Utah), March 26, 1899.

32. "Advice to fat people." *Washington Post*, May 25, 1902, p. 33.

33. "Lost 207 lbs of fat." *Washington Post*, January 19, 1902, p. 12.

34. *Ibid.*

35. Ella Adelia Fletcher. "The effort to appear slender." *Ogden Standard Examiner* (Utah), November 1, 1902.

36. *Ibid.*

37. *Ibid.*

38. W. R. C. Latson, "Methods of reducing obesity." *Los Angeles Times*, September 1, 1903, p. A3.

39. *Ibid.*

40. "Physical culture for stout people." *Elbert County Banner* (Elizabeth, Colorado), February 27, 1903, p. 5.

41. "Exercise for fat people." *Daily Journal* (Telluride, Colorado), March 3, 1903, p. 4.

42. Katherine Morton. "The girl you would like to be." *Salt Lake Herald*, September 11, 1906, p. 22.

43. *Ibid.*

44. *Ibid.*

45. "Too fat and too thin." *Washington Post*, April 10, 1907, p. 6.

46. *Ibid.*

47. "Fat people; thin people." *Ogden Standard Examiner*, May 2, 1907, p. 4.

48. "Fifty ways for fat women to become thin." *Washington Post*, June 16, 1907, p. MS10.

49. *Ibid.*

50. *Ibid.*

51. T. J. Allen. "Daily diet hints." *Washington Post*, June 28, 1910, p. 11.

52. Lina Cavalieri. "My secrets of beauty." *Washington Post*, July 23, 1911, p. M7.

53. *Ibid.*

54. *Ibid.*

55. Lina Cavalieri. "My secrets of beauty." *Washington Post*, October 8, 1911, p. E9.

56. *Ibid.*

57. Lillian Russell. "How to keep from getting fat." *Oakland Tribune*, October 9, 1913.

58. "Work and worry cure obesity." *Los Angeles Times*, January 3, 1913, p. 6.

59. "Fat women should let liquor alone." *Los Angeles Times*, September 17, 1913, sec 2, p. 4.

60. "Has new cure for obesity." *Plateau Voice* (Collbran, Colorado), December 26, 1913, p. 3.

61. "Hints to fat ladies by a great fight trainer." *Los Angeles Times*, December 2, 1913, sec 3, p. 1.

62. Abdul. "Joe Rivers's trainer talks to fat ladies." *Los Angeles Times*, December 3, 1913, sec 3, p. 2.

63. Abdul. "What fat ladies should do after noonday meal." *Los Angeles Times*, December 4, 1913, sec 3, p. 2.

64. "Lemon cure for obesity." *Los Angeles Times*, March 5, 1914, p. 7.

65. "Spinach for the fat guys." *Los Angeles Times*, December 4, 1914, sec 3, p. 1.

66. "Reducing the weight." *Washington Post*, April 11, 1915, p. M2.

67. "How to reduce the weight." *Washington Post*, July 11, 1915, p. MS2.

68. "No bread, no booze in order to get thin, obesity class informed." *Washington Post*, March 5, 1916, p. ES10.

69. Lina Cavalieri. "Summer advice to the fat." *Washington Post*, August 27, 1916, p. MT6.

70. Leonard Keene Hirshberg. "Health and happiness." *Syracuse Herald*, March 21, 1919.

71. "Adequate foods and hints on diet." *New York Times*, October 24, 1909, p. 20.

72. "A word to the fat." *Literary Digest* 51 (October 16, 1915): 837.

Chapter 6

1. "Scraggy people." *Mountain Democrat* (Placerville, California), March 13, 1880.

2. "Fat women's paradise." *Bucks County Gazette* (Pennsylvania), October 11, 1880, p. 7.

3. "American women growing stouter." *Washington Post*, November 2, 1884, p. 4.

4. "The proper weight of man." *The Penn Yan Express* (Penn Yan, New York), November 5, 1884.

5. "Handsome women in Chicago." *Washington Post*, December 14, 1884, p. 7.

6. "A banker robbed by a cowboy." *Liberty Weekly Tribune* (Missouri), November 21, 1884, p. 2.

7. "Society at Cottage City." *New York Times*, July 26, 1885, p. 4.

8. "Fat women." *Decatur Weekly Republican* (Illinois), June 18, 1885, p. 7.

9. Eliza Putnam Seaton. "Fat is the question." *The Galveston Daily News*, April 30, 1899, p. 6.

10. "Pictures of fat women pulled down." *New York Times*, April 7, 1895, p. 16.

11. Katherine Morton. "The girl you would like to be." *Salt Lake Herald*, September 16, 1906, p. 22.

12. "Ladies who are fond of eating savory repasts." *Oakland Tribune*, April 13, 1907, p. 7.

13. "Body weight and vitality." *Washington Post*, September 18, 1908, p. 6.

14. "Why are they fat?" *Syracuse Herald* (New York), September 11, 1911, p. 5.

15. "Call to the fat." *Oakland Tribune*, October 8, 1913.

16. "Thin dresses and fat dresses." *Washington Post*, March 28, 1915, p. D6.

17. Alfred Malsin. "Science turns its attention to stout people." *Washington Post*, April 2, 1916, p. MT5.

Chapter 7

1. Leonard Keene Hirshberg. "Secrets of health and happiness." *Washington Post*, March 27, 1921, p. 52.

2. Winifred Black. "A disgrace to be fat." *Washington Post*, May 23, 1922, p. 9.

3. "Fat women hopeless, says Poiret." *Ogden Standard Examiner* (Utah), January 14, 1923, p. 6.

4. *Ibid.*

5. *Ibid.*

6. "To tax every pound you weigh over 200." *Ogden Standard Examiner* (Utah), February 18, 1923.

7. *Ibid.*

8. Mildred Holland. "Making the most of personality." *Washington Post*, December 20, 1923, p. 11.

9. "Too fat woman a suicide." *New York Times*, January 20, 1927, p. 11.

10. "Toledo bachelor excludes fat women in will." *New York Times*, February 16, 1927, p. 3.

11. "Obesity no cause for divorce, jury in Switzerland decides." *New York Times*, May 1, 1927, p. E6.

12. "Overweight ends life in well." *New York Times*, August 30, 1933, p. 14.

13. "He needed a fat man." *New York Times*, July 17, 1920, p. 4.

14. "Fat women are lazy." *Daily Journal* (Telluride, Colorado), June 1, 1922, p. 1.

15. James C. Young. "Excellent honesty of fat men." *New York Times*, May 13, 1923, p. SM7.

16. "Says nuts are good risks." *New York Times*, November 12, 1924, p. 25.

17. "Fat men are honest." *Washington Post*, September 8, 1927, p. 6.

18. "Fat men are honest, expert holds." *Washington Post*, July 1, 1931, p. 2.

19. "Fat men endure heat better, tests reveal." *Washington Post*, May 6, 1924, p. 2.

20. "Tall children's brains better, says report." *Washington Post*, July 25, 1928, p. 12.

21. "Poor nutrition for the idle warned against." *Washington Post*, June 15, 1935, p. 5.

Chapter 8

1. "Famous fat woman dies." *Washington Post*, March 5, 1922, p. 30.

2. "To tax every pound you weigh over 200." *Ogden Standard Examiner* (Utah), February 18, 1923.

3. "Editor of Nazi paper urges fat folks tax." *Washington Post*, December 14, 1935, p. 9.

4. "305-pound convict wins race of fat men in Sing Sing prison." *New York Times*, September 11, 1922, p. 19.

5. "Trade Board vanquishes dull care at shad frolic." *Washington Post*, May 20, 1923, p. 5.

6. "500 alumni parade in City College fete." *New York Times*, June 15, 1930, p. N3.

7. "Golf and obesity." *New York Times*, January 23, 1921, p. 26.

8. "Fat woman diver sails." *New York Times*, December 17, 1922, p. 21.

9. "Society again out in force at show." *New York Times*, November 17, 1922, p. 23.

10. "Fat men at luncheon." *New York Times*, December 29, 1922, p. 21.

11. "Trade slump lowers tonnage of national fat men's club." *New York Times*, January 21, 1931, p. 20.

12. "Atlanta's police force, 3½ tons overweight." *New York Times*, November 20, 1932, p. E6.

13. "Valentine prefers educated rookies." *New York Times*, December 20, 1938, p. 36.

14. "New policewomen warned on obesity." *New York Times*, March 10, 1939, p. 25.

15. "City holds woman too fat to teach." *New York Times*, July 16, 1935, p. 21.

16. *Ibid.*

17. "In the balance." *Washington Post*, July 25, 1935, p. 8.

18. "180-pound teacher unable to reduce." *New York Times*, August 21, 1935, p. 21; "Wants teachers to be hygienic models." *New York Times*, November 22, 1935, p. 25.

19. "Weight cut to 150, teacher asks job." *New York Times*, December 12, 1935, p. 2.

Chapter 9

1. Leonard Keene Hirshberg. "Secrets of health and happiness." *Washington Post*, March 27, 1921, p. 52.

2. Alonzo E. Taylor. "National overweight." *Washington Post*, April 25, 1931, p. 6.

3. "Stout people inherit fat, says doctor." *Washington Post*, June 22, 1934, p. 14.

4. Logan Clendening. "Today's health talk." *Washington Post*, November 8, 1937, p. 11.

5. "Obesity attacked from mood angle." *New York Times*, April 10, 1938, p. 45.

6. Ida Jean Kain. "Watch your salt and sugar if you want a slender figure." *Washington Post,* June 4, 1938, sec 10, p. 11.

7. Ida Jean Kain. "Your figure madam." *Washington Post*, February 2, 1939, p. 13.

8. Logan Clendening. "Today's health talk." *Washington Post*, July 27, 1939, p. 11.

9. "The perils of fatness." *Literary Digest* 69 (April 2, 1921): 23.

10. W. A. Evans. "How to keep well." *Washington Post*, December 8, 1923, p. 12.

11. "Seekers after death." *Washington Post*, August 26, 1925, p. 6.

12. W. A. Evans. "How to keep well." *Washington Post*, December 17, 1925, p. 14.

13. "Obesity raises death rate." *New York Times*, July 6, 1928, p. 20.

14. "Too many fat people." *Literary Digest* 110 (July 25, 1931): 25.

15. Ida Jean Kain. "Your figure madame!" *Washington Post*, May 1, 1939, p. 11.

Chapter 10

1. "Twenty fat women in reducing course." *New York Times*, April 23, 1920, p. 32.

2. "24 women lose 200 pounds." *Washington Post*, May 7, 1920, p. 6.

3. "The twenty-four against fat, in Chicago." *Literary Digest* 65 (June 5, 1920): 75.

4. "Mobilize fat squad, 50 men, 50 women, in avoirdupois war." *Washington Post*, October 19, 1921, p. 3.

5. "Fat women start long health grind." *New York Times*, October 20, 1921, p. 27.

6. "Fat women getting thin." *New York Times*, October 21, 1921, p. 30.

7. "In training 5 days, can lace her shoes." *New York Times*, October 22, 1921, p. 6.

8. "Fat women lose from 2 to 4 pounds." *New York Times*, October 23, 1921, p. 18.

9. "Fat women are taken on long park hike." *New York Times*, October 24, 1921, p. 12.

10. "Dieting makes two fat women fatter." *New York Times*, October 25, 1921, p. 9.

11. "Police shadow fat women competitors in reducing contest." *Washington Post*, October 27, 1921, p. 3.

12. "Plain clothes women shadow fat women." *New York Times*, October 26, 1921, p. 23.

13. "Pills make a fat contestant fatter." *New York Times*, October 27, 1921, p. 14.

14. "Fair fat reducers balk at taking oil." *New York Times*, October 28, 1921, p. 16.

15. "50 fat women lose 8 feet of waistline." *New York Times*, October 29, 1921, p. 13.

16. "Hundreds write Copeland on fat." *New York Times*, October 30, 1921, p. 35.
17. *Ibid.*
18. "Fat women hike again." *New York Times*, October 31, 1921, p. 8.
19. "481 pounds lost by fifty fat women." *New York Times*, November 1, 1921, p. 11.
20. "Finds fat reducing makes happy homes!" *New York Times*, November 3, 1921, p. 27.
21. "Fat woman gains riding in subway." *New York Times*, November 10, 1921, p. 31.
22. "Fat women close reduction contest." *New York Times*, November 13, 1921, p. 20.
23. "Mayor gives prizes." *New York Times*, November 20, 1921, p. 3.
24. "Fat women hold graduates' reunion." *New York Times*, January 18, 1922, p. 16.
25. "Gains 60 tons of voters." *New York Times*, October 14, 1922, p. 13.
26. "Copeland starts restaurant chain." *New York Times*, October 7, 1925, p. 30.
27. "Women climb 11 flights in trying to cut weight." *Washington Post*, December 17, 1923, p. 8.
28. "Metropolitan's plan for reducing works." *New York Times*, June 26, 1924, p. 38
29. *Ibid.*
30. Louis I. Dublin. "Digging our graves with our teeth." *The Forum and Century* 85 (May, 1931): 314–315.
31. W. A. Evans. "How to keep well." *Washington Post*, July 28, 1924, p. 12.
32. "Fat women busy reducing, thin ones adding weight." *New York Times*, July 26, 1925, sec 10, p. 10.
33. *Ibid.*
34. "Obesity course offered by community center." *Washington Post*, January 24, 1926, p. M6.
35. Viola Paris. "Beauty and you." *Washington Post*, September 4, 1927, p. SM8.
36. "1,200 girl students told what to eat." *New York Times*, December 8, 1927, p. 36.
37. "New diet quickly remedies obesity, doctors informed." *Washington Post*, May 3, 1928, p. 20.
38. "Obesity raises death rates." *New York Times*, July 6, 1928, p. 20.
39. Viola Paris. "Beauty and you." *Washington Post*, August 21, 1928, p. 9.
40. Viola Paris. "Beauty and you." *Washington Post*, August 22, 1928, p. 10.
41. Ruth Ann Davis. "Lecturer gives best methods to cut weight." *Washington Post*, October 9, 1934, p. 13.
42. Orrin E. Dunlap Jr. "Who takes the drills?" *New York Times*, August 19, 1934, sec 20, p. 15.
43. Logan Clendening. "Today's health talk." *Washington Post*, November 8, 1937, p. 11.
44. Ida Jean Kain. "Your figure madam." *Washington Post*, February 2, 1939, p. 13.
45. Ida Jean Kain. "Your figure madame!" *Washington Post*, May 1, 1939, p. 11.
46. Logan Clendening. "Today's health talk." *Washington Post*, July 27, 1939, p. 11.
47. Ida Jean Kain. "Your figure madam." *Washington Post*, December 20, 1939, p. 16.

Chapter 11

1. Mildred Holland. "Making the most of your personality." *Washington Post*, August 16, 1923, p. 10.

2. "Fat women are told how to look slender." *Washington Post*, January 18, 1925, p. A12.

3. Edward T. Folliard. "Sheen of the silver screen." *Washington Post*, April 19, 1925, p. SO13.

4. "Diet experiments are pastime for Hollywood beauties." *Washington Post*, October 29, 1937, p. 17.

5. Virginia Lee Warren. "Plump women languish on fashion's sidelines." *Washington Post*, March 4, 1934, p. 9.

6. "Fall 1940 suits to help fat men look like Gable." *Washington Post*, July 11, 1939, p. 13.

7. "Obesity raises death rates." *New York Times*, July 6, 1928, p. 20.

8. Agnes Lyne. "Guiding your child." *Washington Post*, July 10, 1933, p. 7.

9. Ida Jean Kain. "Your figure madame!" *Washington Post*, July 28, 1939, p. 17.

10. "Fat women hopeless, says Poiret." *Ogden Standard Examiner* (Utah), January 14, 1923, p. 6.

11. W. A. Evans. "How to keep well." *Washington Post*, December 8, 1923, p. 12.

12. "The curse of overweight." *Literary Digest* 91 (November 20, 1926): 25.

13. W. A. Evans. "How to keep well." *Washington Post*, February 5, 1923, p. 10.

14. Louis I. Dublin. "Digging our graves with our teeth." *The Forum and Century* 85 (May, 1931): 311.

15. *Ibid.*, pp. 312–315.

16. "Large waistline held health peril." *New York Times*, August 25, 1933, p. 17.

17. "Weight shortens life of women." *Washington Post*, March 24, 1934, p. 3.

18. Ida Jean Kain. "Your figure madam." *Washington Post*, December 2, 1937, p. 15.

19. Ida Jean Kain. "Your figure madam." *Washington Post*, April 24, 1939, p. 11.

Bibliography

Abdul. "Joe Rivers's trainer talks to fat ladies." *Los Angeles Times*, December 3, 1913, sec 3, p. 2.
_____. "What fat ladies should do after noonday meal." *Los Angeles Times*, December 4, 1913, sec 3, p. 2.
"Adequate foods and hints on diet." *New York Times*, October 24, 1909, p. 20.
"Advice to fat people." *Washington Post*, May 25, 1902, p. 33.
Allen, T. J. "Daily diet hints." *Washington Post*, June 28, 1910, p. 11.
"An awful tale." *Washington Post*, May 31, 1885, p. 4.
"An obesity cure from Europe." *Washington Post*, April 3, 1900, p. 3.
"Angelino tots win ribbons." *Los Angeles Times*, August 5, 1906, p. 18.
"Another way to reduce flesh." *New York Times*, October 8, 1893, p. 18.
"Anti-fat and society women." *Durango Wage Earner* (Colorado), October 26, 1911, p. 3.
"American women growing stouter." *Washington Post*, November 2, 1884, p. 4.
"Appeal to Teutons at Irish bazaar." *New York Times*, October 15, 1916, p. 9.
"Are fat people healthy." *Boulder News and Courier* (Colorado), April 25, 1879, p. 1.
"Are too many fat and lean." *Los Angeles Times*, April 9, 1907, p. 3.
"The art of unfattening." *Brooklyn Eagle*, June 20, 1857, p. 1.
"Atlanta's police force, 3½ tons overweight." *New York Times*, November 20, 1932, p. E6.
"Auxiliary fat men." *New York Times*, February 24, 1877, p. 4.
"A bad county." *Rifle Reveille* (Rifle, Garfield County, Colorado), August 7, 1896, p. 3.
"A banker robbed by a cowboy." *Liberty Weekly Tribune* (Missouri), November 21, 1884, p. 2.
"Baroness Suttner, peace leader, dies." *New York Times*, June 22, 1914, p. 4.
Beacon, Blanche. "Little beauty chats." *Los Angeles Times*, April 14, 1914, sec 2, p. 5.
"Bees buzz and all are happy." *Los Angeles Times*, July 28, 1911, p. 14.
"The big man's year." *Washington Post*, June 17, 1908, p. 17.
"Bingham sued for $100,000." *Washington Post*, June 4, 1910, p. 4.
Black, Winifred. "A disgrace to be fat." *Washington Post*, May 23, 1922, p. 9.
"Body weight and vitality." *Washington Post*, September 18, 1908, p. 6.
Boulder Daily Camera (Colorado), June 17, 1893, p. 2.
"The brigand treatment." *New York Times*, January 6, 1884, p. 6.

Bibliography

"A British disease." *Washington Post*, April 17, 1879, p. 3.
"Call stage heavyweights." *New York Times*, March 1, 1909, p. 9.
"Call to the fat." *Oakland Tribune*, October 8, 1913.
"Catholic picnic." *Los Angeles Times*, August 26, 1897, p. 6.
Cavalieri, Lina. "Mme Cavalieri tells of new obesity treatment." *Washington Post*, January 19, 1913, p. MT7.
_____. "My secrets of beauty." *Washington Post*, July 23, 1911, p. M7.
_____. "My secrets of beauty." *Washington Post*, October 8, 1911, p. E9.
_____. "Summer advice to the fat." *Washington Post*, August 27, 1916, p. MT6.
"Chicago men arrange to have obesity club." *Oakland Tribune*, April 15, 1907, p. 3.
"City holds woman too fat to teach." *New York Times*, July 16, 1935, p. 21.
"The clam gourmands." *New York Times*, August 28, 1874, p. 5.
Clendening, Logan. "Today's health talk." *Washington Post*, November 8, 1937, p. 11.
_____. "Today's health talk." *Washington Post*, July 27, 1939, p. 11.
"A comfort to fat people." *Chester Daily Times* (Pennsylvania), June 21, 1880.
"Consolation for the fat." *Washington Post*, May 24, 1908, p. SM3.
"Copeland starts restaurant chain." *New York Times*, October 7, 1925, p. 30.
"Corpulence and genius." *Washington Post*, March 25, 1914, p. 6.
"Corpulence and sanity." *The Park Record* (Utah), January 13, 1906.
"Corpulency." *Brooklyn Eagle*, April 17, 1863, p. 1.
"The curse of overweight." *Literary Digest* 91 (November 20, 1926): 25.
Daily Journal (Telluride, Colorado), June 28, 1913, p. 1.
Daniels, R. R. "Obesity — its cause and cure." *Box Elder News* (Utah), February 12, 194, p. 6.
Davis, Ruth Ann. "Lecturer gives best methods to cut weight." *Washington Post*, October 9, 1934, p. 13.
"Death from obesity." *Hartford Courant*, September 15, 1853, p. 2.
"The disadvantages of obesity." *Hartford Courant*, May 16, 1891, p. 4.
"Diet experiments are pastime for Hollywood beauties." *Washington Post*, October 29, 1937, p. 17.
"Dieting makes two fat women fatter." *New York Times*, October 25, 1921, p. 9.
"Don't be fat." *Washington Post*, March 24, 1904, p. 8.
"Drink habit." *The Lowell Sun* (Massachusetts), September 23, 1903, p. 5.
Dublin, Louis I. "Digging our graves with our teeth." *The Forum and Century* 85 (May, 1931): 311–316.
Dunlap, Orrin E. Jr. "Who takes the drills?" *New York Times*, August 19, 1934, sec 20, p. 15.
"Editor of Nazi paper urges fat folks tax." *Washington Post*, December 14, 1935, p. 9.
Evans, W. A. "How to keep well." *Washington Post*, February 5, 1923, p. 10.
_____. "How to keep well." *Washington Post*, December 8, 1923, p. 12.
_____. "How to keep well." *Washington Post*, July 28, 1924, p. 12.
_____. "How to keep well." *Washington Post*, December 17, 1925, p. 14.
"The evolution of the corset." *New York Times*, May 11, 1884, p. 11.
"Exercise for fat people." *Daily Journal* (Telluride, Colorado), March 3, 1903, p. 4.
"Fair fat reducers balk at taking oil." *New York Times*, October 28, 1921, p. 16.
"Fake anti-fat cure worries government." *Washington County News* (Utah}, November 26, 1914.
"Fall 1940 suits to help fat men look like Gable." *Washington Post*, July 11, 1939, p. 13.
"Famous fat woman dies." *Washington Post*, March 5 1922, p. 30.
"Fast fat men." *New York Times*, May 25, 1884, p. 3.

Bibliography

"Fasting for corpulent people." *Emery County Progress* (Utah), May 10, 1902.

"Fat and fashionable." *Rocky Mountain News* (Denver), September 18, 1875, p. 3.

"Fat and felony." *Brooklyn Eagle*, July 5, 1865, p. 1.

"Fat and lean people." *The Galveston Daily News*, December 26, 1882.

"The fat and the lean." *Brooklyn Eagle*, April 1, 1887, p. 2.

"Fat as a cure of obesity." *New York Times*, May 2, 1884, p. 2.

"Fat folks turn somersaults." *Aspen Tribune* (Colorado), November 22, 1896, p. 2.

"Fat footpads." *Los Angeles Times*, January 29, 1905, sec 2, p. 8.

"Fat men and jobs." *Los Angeles Times*, October 27, 1907, sec 2, p. 4.

"Fat men are honest." *Washington Post*, September 8, 1927, p. 6.

"Fat men are honest, prison expert holds." *Washington Post*, July 1, 1931, p. 2.

"Fat men are main eventers." *Los Angeles Times*, August 16, 1913, sec 4, p. 2.

"Fat men at luncheon." *New York Times*, December 29, 1922, p. 21.

"Fat men East and West." *San Juan Prospector* (Del Norte, Rio Grand County, Colorado), January 23, 1886, p. 4.

"Fat men eating clams." *New York Times*, September 5, 1879, p. 5.

"Fat men endure heat better, tests reveal." *Washington Post*, May 6, 1924, p. 2.

"Fat men in Put-In-Bay." *Ohio Democrat* (New Philadelphia), August 23, 1872.

"Fat men of genius." *Washington Post*, February 13, 1916, p. S4.

"Fat men on a frolic." *New York Times*, August 24, 1877, p. 8.

"Fat men unpopular now." *Akron Weekly Pioneer Press* (Colorado), April 17, 1914, p. 6.

"The Fat Men's Association." *New York Times*, November 24, 1869, p. 5.

"Fat men's ball." *New York Times*, December 21, 1869, p. 8.

"The fat men's convention." *Richwood Gazette* (Ohio), September 11, 1873.

"Fat people." *Liberty Weekly Tribune* (Missouri), October 6, 1871, p. 1

"Fat people and fluids." *New York Times*, August 22, 1886, p. 10.

"Fat people and fluids." *Brooklyn Eagle*, October 11, 1886, p. 2.

"Fat people blocked traffic on stairs." *Ogden Standard Examiner* (Utah), July 29, 1908.

"Fat people in protest." *The Wasatch Wave* (Utah), August 21, 1908, p. 4.

"Fat people shouldn't wear clothes." *Washington Post*, October 5, 1913, p. MT8.

"Fat people; thin people." *Ogden Standard Examiner* (Utah), May 2, 1907, p. 4.

"Fat woman diver sails." *New York Times*, December 17, 1922, p. 21.

"Fat woman gains riding in subway." *New York Times*, November 10, 1921, p. 31.

"Fat women." *New York Times*, October 6, 1881, p. 4.

"Fat women." *Decatur Weekly Republican* (Illinois), June 18, 1885, p. 7.

"Fat women." *Grand Valley Times* (Utah), December 25, 1896.

"Fat women and thin ones." *Colorado Transcript* (Golden, Jefferson County), August 10, 1898, p. 3.

"Fat women are lazy." *Daily Journal* (Telluride, Colorado), June 1, 1922, p. 1.

"Fat women are taken on long park hike." *New York Times*, October 24, 1921, p. 12.

"Fat women are told how to look slender." *Washington Post*, January 18, 1925, p. A12.

"Fat women busy reducing, thin ones adding weight." *New York Times*, July 26, 1925, p. X10.

"Fat women close reduction contest." *New York Times*, November 13, 1921, p. 20.

"Fat women getting thin." *New York Times*, October 21, 1921, p. 30.

"Fat women hike again." *New York Times*, October 31, 1921, p. 8.

"Fat women hold graduates' reunion." *New York Times*, January 18, 1922, p. 16.

"Fat women hopeless, says Poiret." *Ogden Standard Examiner* (Utah), January 14, 1923, p. 6.

"Fat women lose from 2 to 4 pounds." *New York Times*, October 23, 1921, p. 18.

Bibliography

"Fat women pared down by surgeons." *Oakland Tribune*, June 13, 1908.
"Fat women should let liquor alone." *Los Angeles Times*, September 17, 1913, sec 2, p. 4.
"Fat women start long health grind." *New York Times*, October 20, 1921, p. 27.
"Fat women's paradise." *Bucks County Gazette* (Pennsylvania), October 11, 1880, p. 7.
"50 fat women lose 8 feet of waistline." *New York Times*, October 29, 1921, p. 13.
"Fifty ways for fat women to become thin." *Washington Post*, June 16, 1907, p. MS10.
"Finds fat reducing makes happy homes." *New York Times*, November 3, 1921, p. 27.
"500 alumni parade in City College fete." *New York Times*, June 15, 1930, p. N3.
Fletcher, Ella Adelia. "The effort to appear slender." *Ogden Standard Examiner* (Utah),
    November 1, 1902.
Folliard, Edward T. "Sheen of the silver screen." *Washington Post*, April 19, 1925, p.
    SO13.
"481 pounds lost by fifty fat women." *New York Times*, November 1, 1921, p. 11.
"France may call fat men." *New York Times*, June 21, 1915, p. 2.
"French are gay on Bastille day." *Los Angeles Times*, July 15, 1911, sec 2, p. 3.
"Fruit to reduce flesh." *Washington Post*, December 18, 1898, p. 30
"Fuss of the fat men." *Washington Post*, July 9, 1894, p. 6.
"Gains 60 tons of voters." *New York Times*, October 14, 1922, p. 13.
Garrison, Willard W. "Chicago has 5,000 policemen-athletes. *Kiowa County Press*
    (Eads, Colorado), October 30, 1908, p. 6.
"Gen Shafter on fat men." *Los Angeles Times*, December 9, 1906, sec 7, p. 5.
"The German fat men's target excursion." *New York Times*, June 22, 1870, p. 5.
"Giants and fat men." *New York Times*, March 19, 1905, p. 8.
Gibbs, John Wilson. "Ridding Cleveland of fat." *Salt Lake Tribune*, July 9, 1893, p.
    15.
"The glory of adipose." *New York Times*, August 28, 1884, p. 5.
"A Godsend to all humanity." *Los Angeles Times*, January 29, 1899, p. B5.
"Golf and obesity." *New York Times*, January 23, 1921, p. 26.
"Good word for fat men." *Washington Post*, October 8, 1904, p. 9.
"Grow prosperous: fatten your wife." *Oakland Tribune*, January 4, 1907, p. 14.
"Handsome women in Chicago." *Washington Post*, December 14, 1884, p. 7.
"Has new cure for obesity." *Plateau Voice* (Collbran, Colorado), December 26, 1913,
    p. 3.
"Has new rule for meals." *Washington Post*, April 27, 1914, p. 7.
"He needed a fat man." *New York Times*, July 17, 1920, p. 4.
Herrick, Christine Terhune. "The Times' answers by experts." *Los Angeles Times*, July
    3, 1902, p. A5.
"Hints about health." *Hartford Courant*, September 6, 1888, p. 2.
"Hints for fat persons." *New York Times*, May 14, 1909, p. 11.
"Hints to fat ladies by a great fight trainer." *Los Angeles Times*, December 2, 1913, sec
    3, p. 1.
Hirshberg, Leonard Keene. "Health and happiness." *Syracuse Herald*, March 21, 1919.
_____. "Secrets of health and happiness." *Washington Post*, May 27, 1921, p. 52.
"His baton restored." *Washington Post*, December 5, 1897, p. 3.
Holland, Mildred. "Making the most of personality." *Washington Post*, December 20,
    1923, p. 11.
_____. "Making the most of your personality." *Washington Post*, August 16, 1923, p.
    10.
"Holmes' Star Theater." *Brooklyn Eagle*, August 24, 1890, p. 9.
"Hope for the fat folks." *Hartford Courant*, August 30, 1899, p. 8.

"The housemothers' exchange." *Los Angeles Times*, June 20, 1909, sec 6, p. 2.
"How fat people are made." *Washington Post*, December 26, 1883, p. 2.
"How not to get too fat." *Washington Post*, March 5, 1888, p. 4.
"How to cure obesity." *Washington Post*, November 15, 1885, p. 7.
"How to cure obesity." *Castle Rock Journal* (Colorado), December 30, 1891, p. 3.
"How to get thin." *New York Times*, May 14, 1907, p. 10.
"How to reduce the weight." *Washington Post*, July 11, 1915, p. MS2.
"How stout women may grow thin." *Washington Post*, July 10, 1898, p. 17.
"Human obesity." *The Indiana Democrat* (Indiana, Pennsylvania), August 2, 1883, p. 1.
"Human obesity." *New York Times*, August 18, 1883, p. 3.
"Humorous." *Fort Collins Courier* (Colorado), May 28, 1885, p. 1.
"Hundreds write Copeland on fat." *New York Times*, October 30, 1921, p. 35.
"In the balance." *Washington Post*, July 25, 1935, p. 8.
"In training 5 days, can lace her shoes." *New York Times*, October 22, 1921, p. 6.
"Indebted to our fat men." *San Antonio Daily Light*, November 2, 1888.
"Indict beauty doctors." *New York Times*, June 7, 1912, p. 8.
"Intellect and obesity." *Washington Post*, April 27, 1890, p. 19.
"The jolly fat men of Brooklyn." *New York Times*, December 19, 1869, p. 8.
"Jolly fat men parade." *Washington Post*, September 1, 1893, p. 2.
Kain, Ida Jean. "Watch your salt and sugar if your want a slender figure." *Washington Post*, June 4, 1938, sec 10 p. 11.
_____. "Your figure madam." *Washington Post*, December 2, 1937, p. 15.
_____. "Your figure madam." *Washington Post*, February 2, 1939, p. 13.
_____. "Your figure madam." *Washington Post*, April 24, 1939, p. 11.
_____. "Your figure madam." *Washington Post*, December 20, 1939, p. 16.
_____. "Your figure madame!" *Washington Post*, May 1, 1939, p. 11.
_____. "Your figure madame!" *Washington Post*, July 28, 1939, p. 17.
"Kelp is eaten by Californians as a salad." *Daily Journal* (Telluride, Colorado), March 21, 1898, p. 3.
"Ladies who are fond of eating savory repasts." *Oakland Tribune*, April 13, 1907, p. 7.
"Large waistline held health peril." *New York Times*, August 25, 1933, p. 17.
Latson, W. R. C. "Methods of reducing obesity." *Los Angeles Times*, September 1, 1903, p. A3.
"Laughing makes you fat." *Washington Post*, October 22, 1916, p. MT8.
"Law for fat men." *New York Times*, January 30, 1898, p. 21.
Lee, Ada. "Loses fat — wins fortune." *Washington Post*, April 16, 1912, p. 12.
"Lemon cure for obesity." *Los Angeles Times*, March 5, 1914, p. 7.
"Local matters." *The Union Vedette* (Utah), February 4, 1865, p. 3.
"Lord Rodney, wife beater." *Los Angeles Times*, March 23, 1902, p. A15.
"Lost 207 lbs. of fat." *Washington Post*, January 19, 1902, p. 12.
"A lower berth." *The Oxford Mirror* (Oxford Junction, Iowa), October 4,1883.
Lyne, Agnes. "Guiding your child." *Washington Post*, July 10, 1933, p. 7.
Malsin, Alfred. "Science turns its attention to stout people." *Washington Post*, April 2, 1916, p. MT5.
"Mayor gives prizes." *New York Times*, November 20, 1921, p. 3.
"Metropolitan's plan for reducing works." *New York Times*, June 26, 1924, p. 38.
"Mobilize fat squad, 50 men, 50 women, in avoirdupois war." *Washington Post*, October 19, 1921, p. 3.
"More fat rogues than lean." *Los Angeles Times*, December 23,1906, sec 7, p. 4.

Bibliography

Morton, Katherine. "The girl you would like to be." *Salt Lake Herald*, September 16, 1906, p. 22.

"Most rulers have tendency to fat." *Washington Post*, January 24, 1909, p. E4.

"Motoring spoils figure." *Washington Post*, January 9, 1910, p. A13.

"New diet quickly remedies obesity, doctors informed." *Washington Post*, May 3, 1928, p. 20.

"New policewomen warned on obesity." *New York Times*, March 10, 1939, p. 25.

"No bread, no booze in order to get thin, obesity class is informed." *Washington Post*, March 5, 1916, p. ES10.

"No fat men for football." *New York Times*, March 20, 1905, p. 9.

"No jobs for fat men there." *Lincoln Daily News* (Nebraska), July 1, 196, p. 4.

"No old, short, fat men need apply." *Fort Collins Weekly Courier* (Colorado), April 11, 1906, p. 9.

"Number of fat women is appalling." *Washington Post*, April 25, 1915, p. E14.

"Obesity a bar to office." *New York Times*, February 9, 1916, p. 12.

"Obesity and la grippe." *New York Times*, January 22, 1890, p. 3.

"Obesity attacked from mood angle." *New York Times*, April 10, 1938, p. 45.

"Obesity course offered by community center." *Washington Post*, January 24, 1926, p. M6.

"Obesity no cause for divorce, jury in Switzerland decides." *New York Times*, May 1, 1927, p. E6.

"Obesity raises death rate." *New York Times*, July 6, 1928, p. 20.

"Obesity vs. independence." *Los Angeles Times*, April 8, 1891, p. 7.

"Of interest to fat people." *New York Times*, September 24, 1893, p. 10.

O'Lanus, Corry. "Corry O'Lanus' epistle." *Brooklyn Eagle*, November 27, 1869, p. 2.

"180-pund teacher unable to reduce." *New York Times*, August 21, 1935, p. 21.

"Our quota of club freaks." *Los Angeles Times*, August 1, 1897, p. 17.

"Outing of the Fat Men's Club." *Washington Post*, June 20, 1893, p. 2.

"Overfeeding causes obesity." *Haswell Herald* (Colorado), March 8, 1917, p. 2.

"Overweight ends life in well." *New York Times*, August 30, 1933, p. 14.

Paris, Viola. "Beauty and you." *Washington Post*, September 4, 1927, p. SM8.

_____. "Beauty and you." *Washington Post*, August 21, 1928, p. 9.

_____. "Beauty and you." *Washington Post*, August 22, 1928, p. 10.

"The perils of fatness." *Literary Digest* 69 (April 2, 1921): 23.

"Personal gossip." *Greeley Tribune* (Colorado), October 26, 1893, p. 9.

"Physical culture for stout people." *Elbert County Banner* (Elizabeth, Colorado), February 27, 1903, p. 5.

"Pictures of fat women pulled down." *New York Times*, April 7, 1895, p. 16.

"Pills make a fat contestant fatter." *New York Times*, October 27, 1921, p. 14.

"Plain clothes women shadow fat women." *New York Times*, October 26, 1921, p. 23.

"Platinum cure for obesity." *New York Times*, January 18, 1914, p. C2.

"Police shadow fat women competitors in reducing contest." *Washington Post*, October 27, 1921, p. 3.

"A policeman's happy lot." *New York Times*, June 17, 1882, p. 2.

"Policemen in trouble." *Washington Post*, July 12, 1894, p. 6.

"Poor nutrition for the idle warned against." *Washington Post*, June 15, 1935, p. 5.

"Portly bridal couple." *Los Angeles Times*, December 10, 1911, p. 4.

"The potato habit." *Washington Post*, August 23, 1914, p. M3.

"The proper weight of man." *The Penn Yan Express* (Penn Yan, N. Y.), November 5, 1884.

Bibliography

"Quick lunches make fat men." *Los Angeles Times*, April 25, 1896, p. 14.

"Rather fat." *Brooklyn Eagle*, January 7, 1850, p. 2.

"Reducing the weight." *Washington Post*, April 11, 1915, p. M2.

"Reduction of fat." *The Oxford Mirror* (Oxford Junction, Iowa), November 26, 1886.

"Reduction of obesity." *Los Angeles Times*, August 22, 1913, sec 2, p. 1.

"Risk of great eaters." *The Hillside Standard* (Michigan), August 7, 1866.

Russell, Lillian. "How to keep from getting fat." *Oakland Tribune*, October 9, 1913.

"San Diego County." *Los Angeles Times*, November 30, 1897, p. 13.

"Says fat women pay." *Los Angeles Times*, July 23, 1911, sec 5, p. 20.

"Says nuts are good risks." *New York Times*, November 12, 1924, p. 25.

"Scientific miscellany." *Montezuma Millrun* (Summit County, Colorado), February 25, 1888, p. 3.

"Scraggy people." *Mountain Democrat* (Placerville, California), March 13, 1880.

Seaton, Eliza Putnam. "Fat is the question." *The Galveston Daily News*, April 30, 1889, p. 6.

"Seekers after death." *Washington Post*, August 26, 1925, p. 6.

"She has corset cure." *Washington Post*, February 27, 1908, p. 2.

"She weighs 650 pounds." *Salt Lake Tribune*, March 3, 1889, p. 5.

"Sheridan was third in policemen's games." *New York Times*, August 8, 1906, p. 4.

"Slavery in sweatshops of Paris is revolting." *Oakland Tribune*, April 12, 1908, p. 26.

"Sleep and grow fat." *Hornellsville Tribune* (Steuben County, N. Y.), March 4, 1870, p. 1.

"Smile of fat man sadder than tears." *Oakland Tribune*, May 3, 1908, p. 18.

"Society again out in force at show." *New York Times*, November 17, 1922, p. 23.

"Society at Cottage City." *New York Times*, July 26, 1885, p. 4.

"Some consolation." *Colorado Transcript* (Golden, Jefferson County), December 6, 1893, p. 3.

"Spinach for the fat guys." *Los Angeles Times*, December 4, 1914, sec 3, p. 1.

"Stout parties' picnic." *New York Times*, August 20, 1870, p. 2.

"Stout people inherit fat, says doctor." *Washington Post*, June 22, 1934, p. 14.

"Stout women turned down." *Los Angeles Times*, June 26, 1913, p. 6.

"A talk about freaks." *Brooklyn Eagle*, September 24, 1887, p. 6.

"Tall children's brains better, says report." *Washington Post*, July 25, 1928, p. 12.

"Tapeworm pills for fat people merely a wild yarn, say experts." *Washington Post*, December 6, 1912, p. 5.

Taylor, Alonzo E. "National overweight." *Washington Post*, April 25, 1931, p. 6.

"Ten coppers dropped." *Washington Post*, August 17, 1894, p. 8.

"The terrors of obesity." *Brooklyn Eagle*, November 1, 1885, p. 6.

"Testing a new obesity cure." *New York Times*, September 25, 1898, p. 22.

"The three planes of living." *Literary Digest* 54 (April 7, 1917): 977–978.

"There was fun for everyone." *Los Angeles Times*, August 20, 1911, p. 8.

"Thin dresses and fat dresses." *Washington Post*, March 28, 1915, p. D6.

"Thin fire brigade." *New York Times*, November 22, 1908, p. C4.

"305-pound convict wins race of fat men in Sing Sing prison." *New York Times*, September 11, 1922, p. 19.

"To fat people." *Manti Messenger* (Utah), August 7, 1914, p. 8.

"To reduce one's weight." *Washington Post*, June 2, 1901, p. 23.

"To reduce the abdomen." *Daily Journal* (Telluride, Colorado), August 28, 1901, p. 4.

"To tax every pound you weigh over 200." *Ogden Standard Examiner* (Utah), February 18, 1923.

Bibliography

"To tax fat people." *Breckenridge Bulletin* (Colorado), July 25, 1903, p. 5.

"Toledo bachelor excludes fat women in will." *New York Times*, February 16, 1927, p. 3.

"Too fat and too thin." *Washington Post*, April 10, 1907, p. 6.

"Too fat woman a suicide." *New York Times*, January 20, 1927, p. 11.

"Too many fat people." *Literary Digest* 110 (July 25, 1931): 25.

"Too much for Flushing." *New York Times*, October 9, 1885, p. 3.

"Too solid flesh." *The Rolla New Era* (Missouri), December 26, 1896, p. 4.

"Trade Board vanquishes dull care at shad frolic." *Washington Post*, May 20, 1923, p. 5.

"Trade slump lowers tonnage of national fat men's club." *New York Times*, January 21, 1931, p. 20.

"Traffic officers' field day games." *New York Times*, August 2, 1915, p. 7.

"The true cure of obesity." *Salt Lake Tribune* (Utah), March 26, 1899.

"1,200 girl students told what to eat." *New York Times*, December 8, 1927, p. 36.

"Twenty fat women in reducing course." *New York Times*, April 23, 1920, p. 32.

"The twenty-four against fat, in Chicago." *Literary Digest* 65 (May 7, 1920): 6.

"24 women lose 200 pounds." *Washington Post*, May 7, 1920, p. 6.

"Undue corpulency." *Colorado Transcript* (Golden, Jefferson County), August 2, 1893, p. 7.

"Useful hints to fleshy people." *Liberty Weekly Tribune* (Missouri), June 26, 1885, p. 1.

"Valentine prefers educated rookies." *New York Times*, December 20, 1938, p. 36.

"Value of fruit." *The Rolla New Era* (Missouri), April 23, 1887, p. 4.

"The Victorian obesity." *Leadville Daily and Evening Chronicle* (Colorado), June 5, 1888, p. 1.

"Wants teachers to be hygienic models." *New York Times*, November 22, 1935, p. 25.

Warren, Virginia Lee. "Plump women languish on fashion sidelines." *Washington Post*, March 4, 1934, p. 9.

"Weight cut to 150, teacher asks job." *New York Times*, December 12, 1935, p. 2.

"Weight shortens life of women." *Washington Post*, March 24, 1934, p. 3.

"Were members of the club." *Washington Post*, July 15, 1894, p. 2.

"What car pleases fat men and lean men?" *Los Angeles Times*, September 24, 1916, sec 6, p. 9.

"What determination will do." *Washington Post*, September 29, 1882, p. 2.

Whitaker, Alma. "Are fat men dangerous?" *Los Angeles Times*, December 23, 1913, sec 2, p. 4.

"Why are they fat?" *Syracuse Herald*, September 11, 1911, p. 5.

"Why drinkers are fat." *Littleton Independent* (Colorado), December 31, 1915, p. 6.

"Women climb 11 flights in trying to cut weight." *Washington Post*, December 17, 1923, p. 8.

"A word to the fat." *Literary Digest* 51 (October 16, 1915): 837.

"Work and worry cure obesity." *Los Angeles Times*, January 3, 1913, p. 6.

Young, James C. "Excellent honesty of fat men." *New York Times*, May 13, 1923, p. SM7.

Index

Index

Index

Index